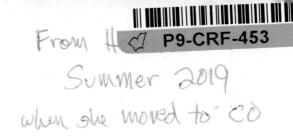

The Sweet Potato Lover's COOKBOOK

More than 100 Ways to Enjoy One of the World's Healthiest Foods

LYNIECE NORTH TALMADGE

Illustrated by Madeleine Watt

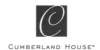

CUMBERLAND HOUSE™

Published by Cumberland House, an imprint of Sourcebooks, Inc.
P.O. Box 4410, Naperville, Illinois 60567-4410
(630) 961-3900
Fax: (630) 961-2168
www.sourcebooks.com

Library of Congress Cataloging-in-Publication Data

Talmadge, Lyniece North.
 The sweet potato lover's cookbook : more than 100 ways to enjoy one of the world's healthiest foods / Lyniece North Talmadge ; Illustrated by Madeleine Watt.
    p. cm.
  Includes index.
 1. Cooking (Sweet potatoes) 2. Cookbooks. I. Watt, Madeleine. II. Title.
   TX803.S94T353 2010
   641.6'522--dc22

                              2010035661

Printed and bound in the United States of America.
CHG 11 10 9 8 7 6

I dedicate this book to my children, Rob and Elizabeth, who encouraged me to write The Sweet Potato Lover's Cookbook *and to my mother, Idella North, who taught me how to cook and to experiment in the kitchen as a child. Cooking and entertaining for my family and friends has given me immense pleasure during the years. I thank Mother, Elizabeth, and Rob for always telling me to "go for it."*

Contents

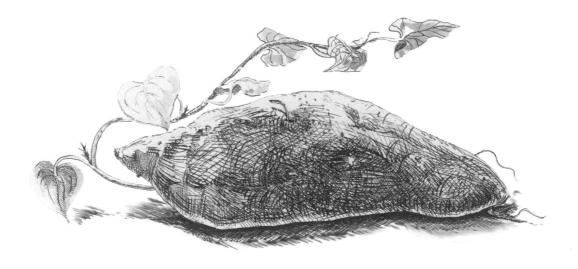

Acknowledgments

There are many people who make a book like this possible. As the author, I had the fun of researching, experimenting, and the tenacious determination to get others to assist in compiling the information on the sweet potato.

First for Madeleine Watt, a talented artist who volunteered to do the outstanding artwork for the book. Madeleine and her family have been friends of mine for over twenty years. Our families have vacationed together on safari in East Africa and shared Thanksgiving holidays at their retreat in North Carolina where we always debated who had the best family recipe for sweet potatoes and who would make the sweet potato dish for the Thanksgiving dinner.

For Lillian and Jack Watt, who have always encouraged me to write something.

For my son, Rob, who taught me to use the computer and researched the Net for me. For all of his tireless encouragement to finish the job as well as for my daughter, Elizabeth, who had no patience with my procrastination.

For Sibley Fleming, a friend and successful author, and Royce Bemis who encouraged me to put the proposal together and begin the job.

For Clio Berney and her parents, Caroline and Richard, who encouraged me.

For the international clients who shared information on sweet potatoes as served in their countries.

For all my guests at Flora Cottage in North Carolina who tried the experimental recipes from soup to dessert—often all at the same meal.

For all my friends who shared recipes in the Friendship chapter.

For Mr. Harold Hoecker, executive secretary of the Sweet Potato Council of the U.S., Inc., who shared recipe information.

For Julie Pitkin and Lisa Taylor and the rest of the staff at Cumberland House whose outstanding efforts helped make *The Sweet Potato Cookbook* come true.

Thank you all for your contributions and belief in me and the book.

The Sweet Potato *story*

It's called the sweet potato. It grows in the ground, is considered a staple in the diet of the lower economic classes, comes wrapped in an ugly brown skin, doesn't stand out among the vast array of supermarket vegetables, and, to be candid, is just plain ugly.

Alas! The lowly sweet potato is an item that is not at the top of the average grocery shopper's list.

But the sweet potato, despite its appearance, is one of nature's unique gifts. It grows throughout the world in the worst of soils and climates, has saved many cultures and civilizations in times of famine, and has been depicted as an honored food in carvings, reliefs, and murals in civilizations such as the Incas, Aztecs, Chinese, Yurubas, and other cultures.

The lowly sweet potato, when eaten, provides the human body with an array of vitamins, minerals, and fiber, and is considered by many professional and amateur athletes to be the quintessential power vegetable. This homely tuber is even being touted as a miracle food that contains strong medicinal potential in fighting an assortment of ailments and diseases. And, if you check with your local health food store, you will find bottles of sweet potato extract, the newly hailed cure-all for everything from the common cold to sexual dysfunction.

These days the sweet potato is at the top of the "new chic foods" list. The Canyon Ranch, one of those ritzy spas that costs $1,000 a day, has started serving fried sweet potatoes in the skin for breakfast. You can bet that the sweet potato will soon be heralded by such notables as Wolfgang Puck and Paula Deen as the new "in" food. It looks like the sweet potato's time has come.

Sweet Potato
facts

- Sweet potatoes and yams are not the same apple: The sweet potato is a vegetable in the morning-glory family Convolvulaceae, while the yam is in the yam family Dioscoreaceae and is grown only in the tropics of western Africa, Southeast Asia, India, and the Caribbean Islands, with a growing season that is too short for the United States.

- A medium size sweet potato weighs about three-fourths of a pound and is considered one serving.

- Sweet potatoes will not turn dark if put in salt water immediately after peeling (1 table-spoon to 1 quart of water).

- Sweet potatoes were cultivated in colonial Virginia in the early 1600s.

- The sweet potato can be either white or yellow, and the yellow sweet potato is grown mostly in the South, while the white sweet potato is grown in Asia and Africa.

- Sweet potatoes have large amounts of Vitamin A and C and are considered one of the top eight high-energy foods by professional athletes. The average sweet potato contains no fat, is only 165 calories, and contains one-half of the daily requirement of Vitamin C and twice the daily requirement of Vitamin A. It is also a terrific source of complex carbohydrates, B vitamins (especially thiamin), protein, iron, calcium, and potassium.

- Every major culture that has survived owes its survival to the sweet potato, including the South after the War Between the States.

- In the late nineteenth century and the early twentieth century, George Washington Carver developed and patented over 118 products made from sweet potatoes and sweet potato by-products.

Sweet Potato
appetizers

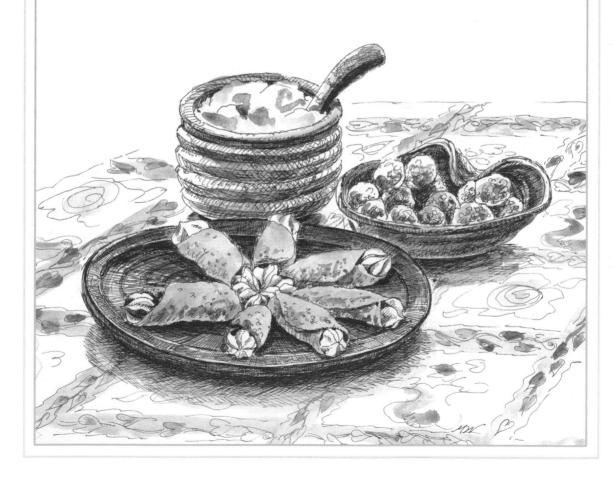

Chips Hors d'Oeuvres

ingredients

2 medium sweet potatoes, scrubbed

Salt to taste

Preheat the oven to 375°. Slice the scrubbed sweet potatoes as thin as possible. I suggest using a mandoline. Place on a cookie sheet sprayed with non-stick cooking spray. Spray the potatoes also. Season with salt to taste. Bake for 35 to 45 minutes.

MAKES ABOUT 30 PIECES

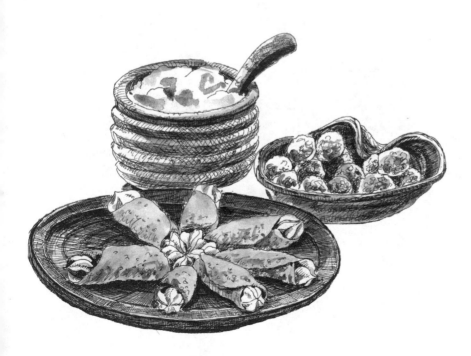

Sweet Potato Phyllo Canapé

ingredients

2 medium sweet potatoes
1 small onion, finely chopped
2 cups finely chopped celery
Olive oil
1 clove garlic, peeled and squashed
Frozen phyllo sheets, thawed
Salt and pepper to taste

Boil the sweet potatoes in a large pot until tender. Cool, then peel by pulling the skin away. Purée in a food processor.

Sauté the onion, celery, and garlic in a skillet wiped with olive oil until the onions are translucent. Remove the garlic clove and add the onion mixture to the sweet potatoes. Blend. Season with salt and pepper.

Preheat the oven to 375°. Peel off a sheet of phyllo according to the directions on the package. Place on a cookie sheet sprayed with a nonstick cooking spray. Fold in half. Place a tablespoon of sweet potato mixture on top and quickly fold over into your favorite shape. Spray with nonstick cooking spray. Do one at a time so the phyllo will not dry out. Bake for 15 to 20 minutes until golden brown and crispy. Serve hot.

MAKES 12 TO 16 SERVINGS

Savory Madeleines

ingredients

2 small sweet potatoes, scrubbed

⅓ cup milk

1 tablespoon unsalted butter, melted

1 egg

Pinch salt and white pepper

Preheat the oven to 400°. Place the sweet potatoes in a saucepan, cover them with water, and bring to a boil. Reduce the heat and simmer about 30 to 40 minutes until tender throughout. Test by spearing a fork into the center. Drain, cool, and peel. Process in a food processor until puréed.

Heat ⅓ cup of milk in the top of a double boiler until tiny bubbles form around the edge of the pan. Add the scalded milk, butter, egg, salt, and pepper to the puréed sweet potatoes and blend.

Spray the madeleine molds with nonstick spray. Spoon the mixture into the molds, filling to the top. Place the madeleine mold pan in the center of the oven. Bake for 20 minutes or until golden brown on the edges. Place the molds on a rack until slightly cooled. Remove the madeleines from the pan and cool completely.

MAKES 16 LARGE OR 40 MINIATURE MADELEINES

For a spicier version, substitute ¼ teaspoon of red pepper for the white pepper.

Buttered Fried Sweet Potatoes

ingredients

3 medium sweet potatoes

5 tablespoons butter

3 to 4 tablespoons balsamic, sherry,
   or red wine vinegar

¼ cup chopped fresh thyme

Salt and pepper to taste

Peel and thinly slice the sweet potatoes crosswise. Melt the butter in a sauté pan or skillet Add the sweet potatoes and sauté over high heat, stirring frequently. While still crunchy, add the vinegar. Stir quickly and season to taste with salt, pepper, and thyme.

MAKES 6 SERVINGS

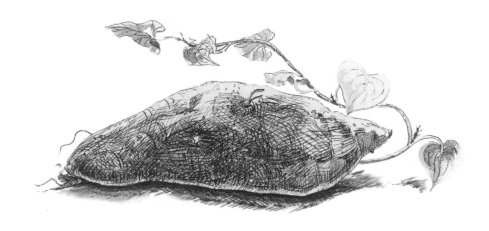

Appetizer Spread

ingredients

1 medium sweet potato

1 tablespoon butter

2 tablespoons milk

1 teaspoon finely chopped fresh
thyme leaves

Preheat the oven to 375°. Wash the sweet potato and spray with vegetable spray. Bake for about 1 hour and 15 minutes until tender.

Scoop out the sweet potato pulp. Combine the pulp, butter, and milk in a food processor, and process until puréed. Fold in the thyme. Use as a spread while still hot.

MAKES ABOUT 6 TO 8 SERVINGS

This is a delicious appetizer served on buttered toasted saltines or toasted pita triangles.

Sweet Potato
beverages

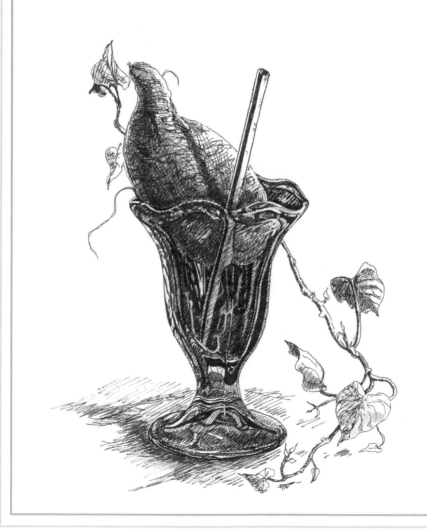

Power Drink

ingredients

1 medium sweet potato

4 stalks celery, stripped and puréed

¼ cup chopped onion

1 (32-ounce) can V-8 juice

Juice of 1 lemon

Salt to taste

Tabasco sauce to taste

Boil the sweet potato in water to cover in a large pot until tender. Peel by pulling the skin away. Purée the sweet potato in a food processor. Add the celery and onion to the processor and blend until evenly mixed. Add the V-8 juice, lemon juice, salt, and Tabasco.

Serve chilled or at room temperature.

Hot Sweet Cinnamon Drink

ingredients

1 medium sweet potato

2 cups apple juice

1 cup orange juice

1 tablespoon firmly packed brown
  sugar

Cinnamon sticks

Freshly grated nutmeg

Boil the sweet potato in water to cover in a large pot until tender. Peel by pulling the skin away. Purée the sweet potato in a food processor. Heat the apple juice, orange juice, brown sugar, and one cinnamon stick in a saucepan until the brown sugar dissolves. Stir in the puréed sweet potato, stirring constantly over low heat until thoroughly blended. Simmer for 2 to 3 minutes.

Pour into mugs and sprinkle grated nutmeg over the top. Add a cinnamon stick to each mug for stirring.

Great for an afternoon pick-me-up or after a cold weather activity.

Southern Punch

ingredients

2 medium sweet potatoes

1 quart boiling water

⅛ teaspoon salt

1½ cups sugar

2 cups pineapple juice

1 (12-ounce) can frozen orange juice concentrate

¼ cup freshly squeezed lemon juice

6 whole cloves

½ teaspoon freshly ground nutmeg

¼ teaspoon cinnamon

¼ teaspoon ground mace

Ginger ale

Orange slices and strawberries

Wash the sweet potatoes and peel. Slice thinly and place in boiling water. Add salt and cook until very tender. Purée the sweet potato slices in a food processor. Return the purée to the water. Combine the sugar, fruit juices, and spices in a saucepan, and bring to a boil. Cook over medium heat for about 10 minutes. Remove the whole cloves. Add the juice mixture to the sweet potato purée. Refrigerate until chilled.

To serve, mix 1 part chilled sweet potato mixture to 3 parts ginger ale. Garnish with orange slices and whole strawberries.

MAKES 1½ GALLONS PUNCH

Sweet Potato *soups*

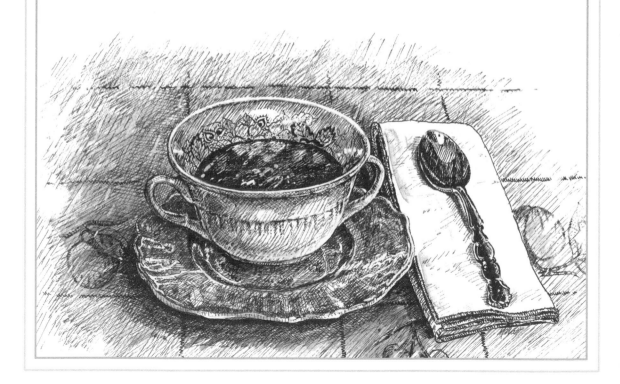

Sweet Potato Soup

ingredients

2 tablespoons margarine

2 onions, chopped

1 celery stalk, diced, plus leaves

2 carrots, peeled and diced

6 cups sweet potatoes, peeled and
   cut into ½-inch pieces

½ to ¾ cup water

2 bay leaves

¼ teaspoon ground nutmeg

¼ teaspoon thyme

1 cup skim milk

Salt and pepper to taste

Heat the margarine and sauté the onions, diced celery stalk, and carrots in a stock pot over low heat. Add the celery leaves and sweet potatoes. Add ½ cup to ¾ cup of water. Add the bay leaves and seasonings. Cover and simmer about 25 minutes until the sweet potatoes are tender.

Discard the bay leaves. Remove the solid vegetables and purée in a food processor. Add back to the stock pot. Add the milk and season with salt and pepper. Simmer over low heat for 15 minutes.

MAKES 6 SERVINGS

Apple and Sweet Potato Soup

ingredients

1 tablespoon butter

1 large onion, minced

2 shallots, minced

4 medium sweet potatoes, peeled
and cubed

2 tart apples peeled, cored, and
cubed

6 carrots, peeled and cubed

1 small papaya, peeled, seeded,
and cubed

1 cup water

3 cups chicken stock

Fresh thyme sprigs

½ cup Crème Fraîche (see page 26)

Melt the butter in a large stock pot and sauté the onion and shallots until limp. Add the sweet potatoes, apples, carrots, and papaya. Reduce the heat and continue cooking for about 10 minutes on low, stirring frequently. Add the water and chicken stock, and simmer on low until the vegetables and fruits are soft. Remove the solid parts of the vegetables and fruits from the soup and purée in a food processor. Return the puréed mixture to the soup and simmer about 10 minutes longer.

Serve hot, garnished with fresh thyme and Crème Fraîche.

Vegetable Sweet Potato Soup

ingredients

3 medium sweet potatoes

1 cup finely chopped onion

2 cloves garlic, peeled and crushed

1 tablespoon olive oil

5 cups beef stock

2 cups finely chopped celery

1 teaspoon finely chopped thyme

1 20-ounce can kidney beans

1 17-ounce can corn

Salt and pepper to taste

Wash the sweet potatoes. Boil in water about 10 minutes until they begin to soften. Drain, peel, and slice. In a stock pot sauté the chopped onion and garlic in olive oil until limp. Add the beef stock, celery, thyme, and sweet potatoes, and bring to a boil. Reduce the heat, cover, and cook for 20 minutes.

Add the kidney beans and corn, and cook 10 minutes more. Season with salt and pepper to taste.

MAKES 8 SERVINGS

Vegetable Stock

ingredients

1 tablespoon sugar

1 tablespoon hot water

Nonstick vegetable cooking spray

3 onions, finely chopped

8 cloves garlic, peeled and crushed

8 sprigs of thyme

6 carrots, peeled and cut into
   1-inch pieces

5 celery stalks, peeled and chopped

4 leeks, cut into 1-inch pieces

4 bay leaves

3 tart apples, quartered

1 onion, studded with 6 whole
   cloves

Celery leaves

Parsley, bunch

½ teaspoon white peppercorns

½ teaspoon black peppercorns

⅛ teaspoon cayenne pepper

Melt the sugar in a small saucepan until it turns dark. Remove from the heat and add the hot water drop by drop to the melted, darkened sugar, stirring constantly. Return to low heat and cook about 3 minutes until a dark liquid. Spray another skillet well with nonstick spray, and sauté the chopped onions until limp. Pour the caramelized sugar, sautéed onions, and all other ingredients into a stock pot, covering with 4 quarts of water. Bring to a boil over medium heat. Reduce the heat and simmer for 2 hours.

Remove from the heat and cool. Strain with a cheesecloth-lined strainer.

MAKES 6 TO 8 CUPS

Lyniece's Soup Stock

ingredients

1 4- to 5-pound baking chicken

5 onions, peeled and quartered

4 carrots, peeled

6 celery stalks, coarsely chopped,
   reserving 1 whole stalk

Celery leaves from bunch

Kosher salt

Lemon pepper

10 garlic cloves, peeled and crushed

6 bay leaves

1 fresh rosemary sprig

4 quarts cold water

½ teaspoon whole peppercorns

8 whole cloves

Parsley, whole bunch

Preheat the oven to 350°. Wash the chicken thoroughly. Scrub all vegetables. Sprinkle a pinch of Kosher salt and lots of lemon pepper inside the cavity of the chicken. Place 4 crushed garlic cloves, 1 quartered onion, 1 bay leaf, rosemary sprig, and 1 celery stalk in the cavity. Place breast side up on a rack in a broiler pan. Bake about 1 hour and 15 minutes until done. Wrap the legs in foil after 45 minutes to prevent overcooking.

Let cool, pull the skin off, and slice the chicken. I use the white meat for sandwiches. Remove the onion, celery, garlic, bay leaf, and rosemary from the cavity. Break apart the carcass. Spoon the liquid oil on top of drippings out of the broiler pan, leaving the crusted brown drippings. Using a wooden spoon, scrape loose the brown drippings and add ½ cup of cold water. Spread the broken carcass and skins around the broiler pan. Cook at 200° for 2 to 3 hours until the bones and skin are brown and crunchy. Scrape everything loose with a wooden spoon and put everything into a heavy stock pot with the cold water. Stud remaining onions with cloves and add to stock pot. Add peppercorns, celery leaves, chopped celery stalks, parsley, remaining bay leaves, remaining garlic, and carrots. Bring to a quick boil and skim the top. Reduce the heat immediately and simmer slowly for 3 hours. Remove from the heat and cool. Strain using a wet cheesecloth-lined strainer. Store the broth airtight in the refrigerator until the fat forms a protective solid mass on top. Leave the fat on top until ready to use. Can be stored like this for 3 to 4 days. The fat can be removed and frozen for later use.

MAKES ABOUT 4 QUARTS

I credit my success with soups to roasting the bones and skin before adding to the stock pot. The sweet potato soups that I make for dinner parties are complimented by all even when they don't like sweet potatoes because the soup started with the best stock, with many layers of taste like a good wine. A medium dry sherry may be added to the finished soup before serving.

Sweet Potato and Greens Soup

ingredients

2 tablespoons margarine

1 cup chopped red onion

2 cloves garlic, minced

6 cups water

1½ cups red lentils, rinsed

3 sweet potatoes, peeled and diced

1 teaspoon fresh ginger, grated

2 teaspoons curry powder

½ teaspoon coriander

¼ teaspoon cinnamon

¼ teaspoon ground nutmeg

6 ounces mustard greens or
   Swiss chard

Juice of 1 lime

Salt to taste

Melt the margarine in a stock pot and sauté the onion and garlic for about 10 minutes. Add the water, lentils, sweet potatoes, and seasonings. Cover and cook on medium heat about 25 to 30 minutes until the sweet potatoes are done.

Wash the greens and remove the hard rib in the center. Cut into small pieces. Stir into the soup with the lime juice and cook until the soup thickens. Reduce the heat and cook about 15 minutes more until the greens are done. Season with salt.

MAKES 6 SERVINGS

Lyniece's Dinner Party Soup

ingredients

4 medium sweet potatoes, baked

Nonstick vegetable spray

8 cups chicken stock

Kosher salt to taste

1 teaspoon orange zest

Nutmeg, freshly grated

3 tart apples, washed and cubed

1 red pepper, cubed

1 yellow pepper, cubed

2 green peppers, cubed

3 cups apple juice

2 tablespoons orange juice
concentrate

Medium dry sherry

1 red and 1 green bell pepper, cut
in strips

Crème Fraîche (see page 26)

Preheat oven to 350°. Wash the sweet potatoes and spray with vegetable spray. Place on a baking sheet and bake for about 1 hour until tender.

Cool, peel, and purée the sweet potatoes and place in a stock pot along with the chicken stock, Kosher salt, orange zest, nutmeg, apple pieces, and cubed red, yellow, and green peppers. Bring to a boil and quickly reduce the heat. Simmer for 20 minutes. Add apple juice and orange juice concentrate, and cook 5 minutes more. Strain. If needed, add a splash of dry sherry to taste. Garnish with red and green pepper strips with a teaspoon of Crème Fraîche.

Tomato Sweet Potato Soup

ingredients

2 medium sweet potatoes

2 large tomatoes

2 carrots

2 stalks celery

2 tablespoons margarine

8 cups beef stock

Salt

Freshly ground white pepper

Crème Fraîche (see page 26)

¼ cup finely chopped scallions

Wash the sweet potatoes. Boil in water about 30 minutes until tender. Drain, cool, peel, and slice. Wash the tomatoes and chop. Wash and grate the carrots in a food processor. String and finely chop the celery. Sauté the carrots and celery in the margarine in a stock pot until limp. Add the beef stock, tomatoes, and sweet potatoes. Bring to a boil, reduce the heat, and simmer for 15 minutes.

Transfer the vegetables to a food processor using a slotted spoon and purée. Return to the stock and simmer for 15 minutes. Season with salt and pepper to taste.

Serve chilled with Crème Fraîche and scallions for garnish.

MAKES 6 TO 8 SERVINGS

Chick Pea and Sweet Potato Soup

ingredients

2 onions, finely chopped

3 cloves garlic, crushed

2 stalks celery, chopped

1 tablespoon olive oil

2 cups canned sweet potatoes,
   drained

3 cups vegetable broth

2 teaspoons paprika

1 teaspoon turmeric

1½ cups canned chick peas, drained

1 cup chopped green bell pepper

2 bay leaves

1 teaspoon basil

2 cups chopped tomatoes

Freshly ground black pepper

Dash Tabasco sauce

2 teaspoons Worcestershire sauce

3 tablespoons sour cream for
   garnish

In a stock pot sauté the onion, garlic, and celery in the olive oil for 4 minutes. Add everything except the Tabasco and Worcestershire sauces. Bring to a boil. Reduce the heat and simmer for 15 minutes. Add the Tabasco and Worcestershire sauces to taste. Garnish with a spoonful of sour cream.

MAKES 6 SERVINGS

Andouille Sausage and Sweet Potato Soup

ingredients

5 medium sweet potatoes

1 pound Andouille sausage

2 red peppers

2 yellow peppers

2 green peppers

5 cups chicken stock

1 cup concentrated apple juice

1 teaspoon grated orange rind

3 tablespoons tomato paste

1 bay leaf

Boil the sweet potatoes in a large pot in water to cover until tender. Drain, cool, peel, and coarsely mash. Partially cook the sausage in a skillet. Wipe off the excess fat after cooking. Wash, core, and thinly slice the peppers. Combine the chicken stock, apple juice, sweet potatoes, orange rind, and tomato paste in a stock pot. Reserve 8 strips each of red, yellow, and green pepper for garnish. Add the remaining peppers to the stock pot. Stir well until blended on medium heat. Add the bay leaf and sausage and simmer for 35 minutes. Discard the bay leaf.

MAKES 4 SERVINGS

This dish reminds me of New Orleans. It is great with a baguette.

Vidalia Onion and Sweet Potato Soup

ingredients

2 cups canned sweet potatoes

2 tablespoons olive oil

3 Vidalia onions (1 chopped and
   2 thinly sliced)

3 cups chicken stock

Salt and pepper to taste

¾ cup heavy cream

Crème Fraîche (see page 26)

Drain the sweet potatoes and purée in a food processor. Heat the olive oil in a skillet and sauté the chopped onion until limp. Combine the sweet potatoes, sautéed onion, and chicken stock in a stock pot and bring to a boil. Immediately reduce the heat and simmer for 20 minutes.

Add the salt, pepper, and cream, and blend well. Remove from the heat and ladle into hot soup plates. Top with Vidalia onion rings and Crème Fraîche.

MAKES 4 SERVINGS

Yellow Split Pea Soup and Spiced Yogurt

ingredients

2 tablespoons clarified butter
   or 1 tablespoon olive oil and
   1 tablespoon regular butter
1 large yellow onion, diced
2 cloves garlic, minced
1 1-inch piece fresh ginger root,
   peeled and minced
1 bay leaf
1 teaspoon salt
½ teaspoon cumin
3 whole cloves
1⅔ cups yellow split peas, soaked
   for 2 hours or longer
1 celery heart, diced
2 medium sweet potatoes, peeled
   and cut
7 cups water or stock
Salt to taste
Grated peel and juice of 1 lemon
Spiced Yogurt
Cilantro or parsley, chopped, for
   garnish

Spiced Yogurt
½ cup plain yogurt
½ teaspoon turmeric
½ teaspoon paprika
¼ teaspoon cayenne pepper
¼ teaspoon cumin
Pinch salt

Heat the clarified butter in a stock pot and add the onion, garlic, ginger, bay leaf, and salt. Grind the cumin seeds and cloves in a spice mill and add to the onion mixture. Stir everything together and cook for 4 minutes.

Drain the peas and add to the onion mixture with the celery, sweet potatoes, and water or stock. Bring to a boil, reduce the heat, and simmer for 45 to 60 minutes until the peas have fallen apart.

Pass through a blender and return to the stove. Add more stock as needed. Season with salt, lemon peel, and lemon juice.

Serve with Spiced Yogurt and a sprinkling of cilantro.

To make the Spiced Yogurt

Combine the yogurt, turmeric, paprika, cayenne, cumin, and salt in a small bowl. Whisk together until smooth.

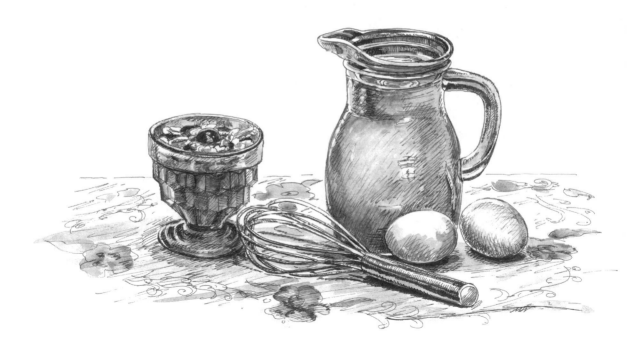

Butter Pecan Soup

ingredients

Crème Fraîche

1 cup heavy cream

1 cup sour cream

Soup

2 tablespoons unsalted butter

¾ cup finely chopped onion

1 cup finely chopped leek

2 large cloves garlic, minced

2 large carrots, thinly sliced

1 bay leaf

Salt and pepper to taste

3 large sweet potatoes

1 baking potato

4 cups chicken broth

1 cup water, or as needed

1 cup white wine

Topping

¾ cup chopped pecans

2 tablespoons unsalted butter

To make the Crème Fraîche

Combine the cream and sour cream in a saucepan. Mix well and heat over low heat until warm. Put into a covered jar and let sit at room temperature for 6 to 8 hours. Refrigerate overnight before using. Keeps 2 to 3 weeks.

MAKES ABOUT 2 CUPS

To make the Soup

Melt the butter and sauté the onion, leek, garlic, and carrots in a stock pot until the onion is tender. Add the bay leaf, salt, and pepper. Peel and very thinly slice the sweet potatoes and baking potato. Add the chicken broth, water, and potatoes to the stock pot. Bring almost to the boiling point. Reduce the heat and simmer for 30 minutes or until the potatoes are tender. Transfer to a blender and purée the mixture until smooth. Return to the pot with the wine. Simmer 10 minutes more.

To serve, pour into soup plates and place pecans and Crème Fraîche in the center.

MAKES 6 TO 8 SERVINGS

To make the Topping

Toast the pecans in butter in the oven at 300° for about 10 minutes.

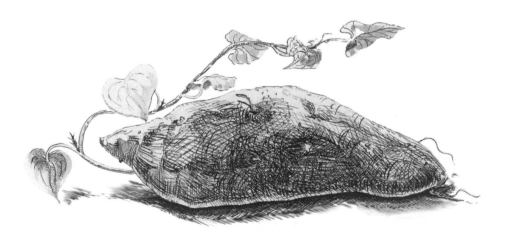

Peanut–Sweet Potato Soup

ingredients

3 medium sweet potatoes

1 tablespoon butter

2 tablespoons minced shallots
  or onion

2 cups thick pumpkin purée

8 cups chicken broth

1 cup pure, unsalted peanut butter

2 teaspoons dry mustard

½ teaspoon nutmeg

Salt and white pepper to taste

Fresh chives

Preheat the oven to 350°. Place the sweet potatoes on a baking sheet. Bake for 1 hour.

Cool and peel the sweet potatoes. Purée the peeled sweet potatoes in a food processor. Measure out 2 cups and set aside.

Melt the butter over medium heat in a large heavy pot. Add the shallots or onion and sauté for 2 minutes. Add the reserved processed potatoes and the pumpkin purée. Alternately add the broth and peanut butter, stirring the mixture after each addition. Bring the soup to a boil. Reduce the heat and simmer for 25 minutes.

Stir in the mustard, nutmeg, salt, and pepper. Before serving, garnish with chives.

Can be made several days ahead and frozen.

MAKES 8 TO 12 SERVINGS

Chilled Curried Soup

ingredients

1 tablespoon vegetable oil

3 medium sweet potatoes, peeled
   and thinly sliced

1 onion, thinly sliced

1 teaspoon curry powder

2 cups chicken broth

4 cups water

Fresh chives, chopped

Heat the oil in a stock pot and sauté the thinly sliced sweet potatoes and onion over moderately low heat, stirring occasionally, until onion and sweet potatoes are limp. Add the curry powder, stir, and cook for 3 minutes more. Add the broth and water. Bring just to a boil, reduce the heat, and simmer for 25 minutes or until the sweet potatoes are tender.

Transfer the mixture to a food processor and purée until smooth. Cool immediately, cover, and chill until cold.

Garnish with fresh chives. May be prepared the day before.

MAKES 4 TO 6 SERVINGS

Sweet Potato Bisque

ingredients

2 ribs celery, trimmed and chopped

2 medium onions, peeled and chopped

3 medium sweet potatoes, peeled and chopped

4 cups water

4 beef bouillon cubes

1 bay leaf

1½ teaspoons tarragon

2 cups milk, scalded

Salt and pepper to taste

Chopped parsley

Combine the celery, onions, sweet potatoes, water, bouillon cubes, bay leaf, and tarragon in a soup pot, and bring to a boil. Reduce the heat and simmer for 30 minutes until tender.

Purée the mixture in a food processor. Return to the pot and add the scalded milk. Season with salt and pepper. Garnish with parsley.

MAKES 8 TO 10 SERVINGS

Georgia Sweet Potato Soup

ingredients

3 tablespoons margarine or
  unsalted butter

2 Vidalia onions, finely chopped

4 medium sweet potatoes, peeled
  and chopped

2 Golden Delicious apples, peeled
  and chopped

5 cups vegetable or chicken stock

1½ cups apple juice

¼ teaspoon freshly grated nutmeg

⅛ teaspoon cinnamon

⅛ teaspoon allspice

Salt and pepper to taste

Melt the margarine in a stock pot and sauté the onions until translucent. Add the chopped sweet potatoes and apples, and cook for 2 to 4 minutes. Add half of the stock and bring to a boil. Reduce the heat and simmer for 30 minutes.

Purée the mixture in a food processor until smooth. Return the mixture to the pot and add the remaining stock, apple juice, and spices. Season with salt and pepper. Cook over low heat until hot.

Serve hot with apple or cinnamon garnish.

Fennel and Sweet Potato Soup

ingredients

2 tablespoons margarine

3 medium sweet potatoes, peeled
   and chopped

½ large fennel bulb, sliced

1 large onion, finely chopped

6 cups chicken stock

1 tablespoon nondairy creamer

1 tablespoon lemon juice

Dill sprigs

Lemon slices

Melt the margarine in a stock pot and sauté the sweet potatoes, fennel, and onion until the onion is translucent. Add the chicken stock and bring to a boil. Reduce the heat and cook over low heat until the vegetables are soft.

Purée the mixture in a food processor until smooth. Return the mixture to the pot. Add the creamer and lemon juice. Reheat until hot and serve. Garnish with dill sprigs and a lemon slice.

Sweet Potato *salads*

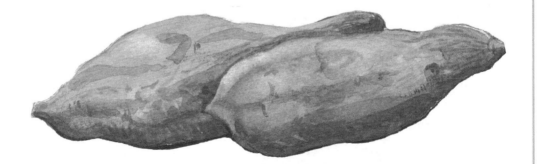

Hawaiian Salad

ingredients

3 medium sweet potatoes

1 tablespoon lemon juice

1 cup pineapple chunks with juice

¼ to ⅓ cup light mayonnaise

1 cup peeled and sliced celery

Romaine lettuce leaves

Wash and peel the sweet potatoes. Cut into 1-inch cubes and place in a vegetable steamer over boiling water. Steam about 10 to 15 minutes until done. The sweet potatoes must still be firm. Cool the sweet potatoes and sprinkle with lemon juice. Drain the pineapple chunks, reserving 1 tablespoon of pineapple juice. Mix the pineapple juice with the mayonnaise in a small bowl to make the dressing. Toss the sweet potato chunks, pineapple chunks, celery, and mayonnaise-pineapple juice dressing in a large bowl until well coated.

Serve on a bed of crisp heart of Romaine lettuce leaves.

MAKES 6 TO 8 SERVINGS

New Orleans Salad

ingredients

6 medium sweet potatoes

5 scallions, finely chopped

2 yellow bell peppers, sliced in strips

2 red bell peppers, sliced in strips

1 green bell pepper, sliced in strips

Dressing

¼ cup red wine vinegar

1 tablespoon sugar

⅓ cup Dijon mustard

Dash cayenne pepper

Kosher salt

½ cup olive oil

Wash and peel the sweet potatoes. Cut into 1-inch cubes and place in a vegetable steamer over boiling water. Steam about 10 to 15 minutes until done. The sweet potatoes must still be firm. Cool the sweet potatoes. Combine the chopped scallions, including the tops, and the peppers with the sweet potatoes in a large bowl. Set aside and make the dressing.

Mix together the red wine vinegar, sugar, and Dijon mustard in a food processor. Add the Kosher salt and cayenne pepper to taste. With the food processor on, pour the olive oil into the dressing mixture and process until well blended.

Toss the salad with the dressing until well coated.

MAKES 6 TO 8 SERVINGS

Waldorf Sweet Potato Salad

ingredients

4 medium sweet potatoes

4 baking apples

2 tablespoons lemon juice

2 tablespoons sugar

2 tablespoons golden raisins

3 tablespoons chopped walnuts

¼ teaspoon salt

Dressing

¼ cup plain nonfat yogurt

2 tablespoons light mayonnaise

Wash and peel the sweet potatoes. Cut into 1-inch cubes and place in a vegetable steamer. Steam over boiling water about 10 to 15 minutes until done. The sweet potatoes must still be firm. Cool the sweet potatoes. Scrub the apples, core, and cut into 1-inch cubes. Sprinkle the apples with lemon juice and sugar.

Combine the raisins, walnuts, salt, sweet potatoes, and apples in a large bowl. Mix together the yogurt and mayonnaise in a small bowl to make the dressing.

Toss the dressing with the sweet potato and apple mixture.

MAKES 6 TO 8 SERVINGS

Sweet Potato Salad

ingredients

6 unpeeled sweet potatoes

1 small onion, diced

1 rib celery, diced

½ cup chopped fresh parsley

2 tablespoons olive oil

2 tablespoons fresh lemon juice

2 teaspoons soy sauce

1 teaspoon marjoram

Freshly ground black pepper

½ cup unsalted roasted cashews

Cover the sweet potatoes in water in a large pot and bring to a boil. Reduce the heat and simmer for 30 minutes until tender. Remove from the water and peel. Chill and then cut into cubes.

Combine the sweet potatoes, onion, celery, and parsley in a large bowl. Combine the olive oil, lemon juice, soy sauce, marjoram, and pepper in a jar.

Pour over the potato mixture, tossing lightly. Garnish with cashews.

MAKES 6 SERVINGS

Slim and Smart Salad

ingredients

½ cup low fat cottage cheese

1 tablespoon plain low fat yogurt

1 tablespoon Dijon mustard

½ teaspoon balsamic vinegar

⅛ teaspoon sugar

2 cups cooked ham, cut in strips

2 cups peeled and diced cooked
  sweet potatoes

2 large stalks celery, thinly sliced

Blend the cottage cheese, yogurt, Dijon mustard, balsamic vinegar, and sugar in a blender or food processor at high speed for about 20 seconds. Combine the ham, sweet potatoes, and celery in a large bowl. Pour the dressing over and toss gently to mix.

The dressing can be refrigerated in a covered container up to 24 hours.

MAKES 4 SERVINGS

—*Sweet Potato Council of the U.S., Inc.*

Sweet Potato *breads*

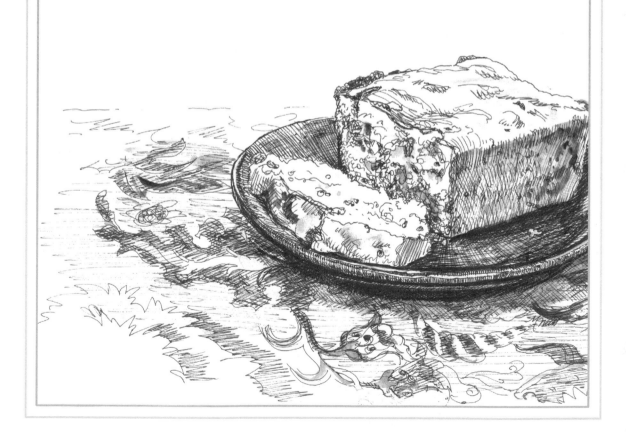

Apple Sweet Potato Bread

ingredients

3 cups all-purpose flour

¼ teaspoon salt

2 teaspoons baking soda

1½ teaspoons cinnamon

1 teaspoon freshly grated nutmeg

1 teaspoon ground cloves

¼ teaspoon allspice

2 cups canned sweet potatoes

¾ cup vegetable oil

2 cups sugar

4 large eggs, beaten

2 tart apples, peeled and chopped

Topping

1 tablespoon all-purpose flour

¼ cup sugar

1 teaspoon cinnamon

1 tablespoon unsalted butter

Preheat the oven to 350°. Spray two 9x5x3-inch loaf pans with vegetable spray. Sift together 3 cups of flour, salt, baking soda, 1½ teaspoons of cinnamon, nutmeg, cloves, and allspice in a medium bowl. Mix together the sweet potatoes, oil, 2 cups of sugar, and eggs in a separate bowl until well blended. Fold in the apples. Add the dry ingredients, stirring just enough to blend. Divide the batter among the two loaf pans.

To make the Topping

Blend 1 tablespoon of flour, ¼ cup of sugar, 1 teaspoon of cinnamon, and butter together until it resembles coarse meal. Sprinkle on top of the batter. Bake about 45 minutes until done.

The bread is done when a toothpick inserted in the center comes out clean. Cool in the pans. May be frozen.

MAKES 2 LOAVES

Sweet Potato Oat Bran Biscuits

ingredients

1¼ cups all-purpose flour

1 tablespoon baking powder

¼ teaspoon salt

2 tablespoons firmly packed
    brown sugar

1 cup oat bran

¼ cup butter, chilled

¼ cup low fat milk

1 large cooked sweet potato,
    mashed

Preheat the oven to 425°. Sift together the flour, baking powder, and salt in a large bowl. Stir in the brown sugar and oat bran. Cut in the butter with a pastry blender until the mixture resembles coarse crumbs. Stir in the milk and sweet potato, making a soft dough. Knead the dough lightly on a floured board until smooth. Roll out ½-inch thick. Cut into rounds. Place on a greased baking sheet. Bake for about 15 to 18 minutes or until browned.

MAKES ABOUT 18 BISCUITS

Sweet Potato Biscuits

ingredients

2 cups cooked, mashed sweet
  potatoes

6 tablespoons butter

1 tablespoon sugar

1½ cups all-purpose flour

½ cup whole wheat flour

4 teaspoons baking powder

½ teaspoon salt

Combine the sweet potatoes, 3 tablespoons of butter, and the sugar in a large bowl. Combine the flours, baking powder, and salt in a small bowl. Add the flour mixture to the sweet potato mixture, stirring until combined into a dough.

Preheat the oven to 375°. Roll the dough out ½-inch thick on a floured board. Using a floured biscuit cutter, cut out the biscuits and place on a greased baking sheet. Brush the biscuits with the remaining butter. Bake for 20 minutes or until the tops are lightly browned.

MAKES 20 BISCUITS

Sweet Potato Pancakes

ingredients

1 cup all-purpose flour

1 teaspoon baking powder

2 tablespoons sugar

⅛ teaspoon ground cinnamon

⅛ teaspoon ground cloves

⅔ cup cooked and puréed sweet
   potato

1 tablespoon butter, melted

1 cup milk

1 egg, beaten

Maple syrup or fruit syrups

Combine the flour, baking powder, sugar, cinnamon, and cloves in a large bowl. Combine the sweet potato and butter in a separate bowl, stirring well. Gradually stir in the milk and beaten egg. Add to the dry ingredients, stirring until moistened. Spoon 2 tablespoons of batter onto a hot, lightly greased griddle. Turn the pancakes when the tops are covered with bubbles and the edges are brown.

Serve with maple syrup or any fruit syrups.

MAKES 1 DOZEN PANCAKES

Orange Butter Sweet Potato Waffles

ingredients

1¾ cups canned sweet potatoes, drained

2¼ cups all-purpose flour

4 teaspoons baking powder

1 teaspoon salt

4 eggs

4 tablespoons margarine, melted

⅓ cup firmly packed brown sugar

2 tablespoons freshly grated orange rind

Low fat milk

Honey

Orange Butter

½ cup butter, softened

3 tablespoons freshly grated orange rind

⅛ teaspoon freshly grated nutmeg

Purée the drained sweet potatoes in a food processor. Sift together the flour, baking powder, and salt in a medium bowl. Beat the eggs in a large bowl until fluffy. Add the puréed sweet potatoes to the beaten eggs. Add the melted margarine, brown sugar, and grated orange rind, mixing well. Add the dry ingredients and blend. If the batter is too stiff, add a few drops of low fat milk to reach the right consistency. Spray a heated waffle iron with nonstick spray. Pour ¾ to 1 cup of batter into the waffle iron and cook until done. Repeat. Serve with Orange Butter and honey.

To make the Orange Butter

Whip the butter in a medium bowl until light and creamy. Blend in the orange rind and nutmeg.

MAKES 6 WAFFLES

Sweet Potato Corn Sticks

ingredients

2 medium sweet potatoes

1 cup yellow cornmeal

1 cup unbleached all-purpose flour

½ cup sugar

2½ teaspoons baking powder

½ teaspoon salt

2 eggs

6 tablespoons butter

½ cup buttermilk

Preheat the oven to 400°. Boil the sweet potatoes in a large pan in water to cover until tender. Drain, cool, and peel. Purée the sweet potato in a food processor. Measure 1½ cups of the purée. Spray a cast-iron corn stick pan with vegetable spray and heat until the pan smokes. Combine the cornmeal, flour, sugar, baking powder, and salt in a medium bowl. Mix together the sweet potatoes, eggs, butter, and buttermilk in a large bowl. Stir the dry ingredients into the potato mixture. Spoon the batter into the hot pans, filling each three-fourths full. Bake for 15 to 20 minutes.

Cool in the pans for 5 minutes before serving.

MAKES 12 TO 14 STICKS

Sweet Potato Corn Bread

ingredients

1 medium sweet potato, peeled
   and quartered

½ cup butter, softened

¾ cup firmly packed brown sugar

4 eggs

1 cup milk

½ teaspoon salt

2 cups white cornmeal

Boil the sweet potato in salted water in a large pot until tender. Drain and mash. Preheat the oven to 400°. Butter a shallow 10x14-inch baking pan. With an electric mixer, cream together the butter and brown sugar until light. Beat in the eggs, one at a time. Beat in the sweet potato, milk, and salt. Stir in the cornmeal until the batter is combined. Pour into the prepared pan and bake about 30 minutes until firm. Serve hot.

MAKES 6 TO 8 SERVINGS

Indian Sweet Potato Corn Bread

ingredients

3 small or 2 medium sweet
  potatoes

1 cup cornmeal

½ teaspoon salt

2 teaspoons baking powder

1 cup water or milk

Preheat the oven to 375°. Place the sweet potatoes in a small baking pan and bake about 1 to 1½ hours until tender. Cool briefly, scoop out, and mash the pulp. Measure 2 cups of pulp. Butter a 10-inch round cake pan. Stir together the cornmeal, salt, and baking powder in a large bowl. Add the water or milk. Stir in the mashed potatoes. Spoon into the prepared pan. Bake for 30 to 40 minutes until firm.

MAKES 6 SERVINGS

Cornmeal Sweet Potato Muffins

ingredients

¾ cup all-purpose flour

2½ teaspoons baking powder

½ teaspoon baking soda

¾ teaspoon salt

1 cup yellow cornmeal

1 cup buttermilk

2 eggs, beaten lightly

2 cups puréed canned sweet
potatoes

2 tablespoons unsalted butter,
melted

Preheat the oven to 400°. Sift together the flour, baking powder, baking soda, salt, and cornmeal in a large bowl. Combine the buttermilk, eggs, sweet potatoes, and melted butter in a separate mixing bowl. Gradually add the sweet potato mixture to the dry ingredients, stirring just enough to blend.

Spoon the batter into a muffin pan coated with a vegetable spray, filling cups three-fourths full. Reduce the heat to 375° and bake in the middle of the oven for 25 minutes or until done.

MAKES 24 MUFFINS

Hahira Muffins

ingredients

1 cup canned sweet potatoes

2 cups sifted all-purpose flour

2 teaspoons baking powder

½ teaspoon salt

½ teaspoon ginger

½ teaspoon freshly ground nutmeg

⅛ teaspoon ground cloves

⅓ cup raisins

¾ cup firmly packed brown sugar

⅓ cup butter, softened

¼ cup molasses

½ cup milk

2 eggs, beaten

Preheat the oven to 375°. Drain the sweet potatoes and mash. Sift together the flour, baking powder, salt, and spices in a medium bowl. Add the raisins and coat with the flour mixture. Cream the brown sugar, butter, and molasses in a large bowl. Add the milk, eggs, and mashed sweet potatoes, blending well. Stir in the dry ingredients, blending only until the flour disappears.

Spray 12 muffin cups with vegetable spray. Fill the muffin cups with batter. Bake for 16 to 18 minutes.

MAKES 12 LARGE MUFFINS

Sweet Potato Muffins

ingredients

1 large sweet potato

1 cup all-purpose flour

1 teaspoon baking powder

¼ teaspoon baking soda

½ teaspoon salt

½ teaspoon ground cinnamon

½ teaspoon ground nutmeg

1 egg, beaten

¼ cup milk

¼ cup sugar

½ cup chopped pecans

Preheat the oven to 350°. Boil the sweet potato in water to cover until tender. Drain, cool, and peel. Transfer to a food processor and purée. Sift together the flour, baking powder, baking soda, salt, cinnamon, and nutmeg in a medium bowl. Mix the egg, sweet potato purée, milk, and sugar in a large bowl. Add the sifted dry ingredients to the liquid mixture, blending well. Add the chopped pecans and mix well.

Spray a muffin pan with vegetable spray. Bake for 25 minutes. Cool and remove from the muffin pan.

Sweet Potato Butter Spread

ingredients

1 medium sweet potato

1 cup unsalted butter, softened

Freshly grated nutmeg

Wash the sweet potato and boil in water about 30 minutes until tender. Drain, cool, and peel. Purée the sweet potato in a food processor. Add the butter and pulse until smooth. Add the nutmeg.

MAKES ABOUT 1½ CUPS OF SPREAD

Great to serve with fresh bread. My son, Rob, introduced this spread to me, and I now serve it with fresh bread and a bowl of soup for lunch.

Sweet Potato Cheese Bread

ingredients

1 17-ounce can sweet potatoes

2½ cups sugar

1 8-ounce package cream cheese

½ cup margarine

4 eggs

3½ cups flour

2 teaspoons baking soda

1 teaspoon salt

1 teaspoon cinnamon

½ teaspoon ground cloves

1 cup chopped pecans

Preheat the oven to 350°. Drain the sweet potatoes and purée. Combine the sugar, cream cheese, and margarine in a large bowl, mixing until well blended. Add the eggs one at a time, mixing well after each addition. Add the sweet potato purée and blend well. Combine the flour, baking soda, salt, cinnamon, and cloves in a separate bowl, and sift into the sweet potato mixture. Fold in the pecans. Spray two 9x5-inch loaf pans with nonstick spray. Pour the mixture into the loaf pans. Bake for 1 hour or until a wooden toothpick inserted into the center comes out clean.

Cool for ten minutes before removing from the pans.

MAKES 2 LOAVES OR 24 SLICES

Sweet Potato Cloverleaf Rolls

ingredients

1 sweet potato, cubed

Reserve ¼ cup cooking water
   from sweet potatoes

½ cup nonfat dry milk

2 tablespoons firmly packed
   brown sugar

2 tablespoons unsalted butter at
   room temperature, in ½ inch pieces

¾ teaspoon Kosher salt

2 cups bread flour

1 teaspoon active dry yeast, instant
   or bread machine

Milk for brushing tops of rolls

Place the cubed sweet potatoes in a saucepan with water to cover by 1 inch. Bring to a boil, then reduce heat and simmer until potatoes are tender, about 15 to 20 minutes. Drain, reserving ¼ cup of cooking water. Purée sweet potatoes.

Place ½ cup puréed sweet potatoes, cooking water, nonfat dry milk, brown sugar, butter, salt, bread flour, and yeast in baking pan fitted with kneading paddle. Press "menu" and select "dough/pizza dough." Select "1 lb." dough size. Press "start" to mix, knead, and rise. When dough is ready, remove from baking pan and deflate. Divide into nine equal portions. Lightly coat nine-hole muffin tin with cooking spray. Divide each dough ball into three equal pieces. Roll each piece into a small ball. Arrange three small dough balls in each muffin cup. Cover with plastic wrap and let rise until doubled, about 30 to 40 minutes. Preheat oven to 375°. When rolls have doubled in size, brush tops with milk. Bake in preheated oven for 20 to 25 minutes, until lightly browned and hollow sounding when tapped. Remove from muffin tins and serve warm. May be made ahead and reheated to serve.

1 POUND OF DOUGH WILL PRODUCE 8 ROLLS

Use a convection bread maker.

Sweet Potato
breakfasts

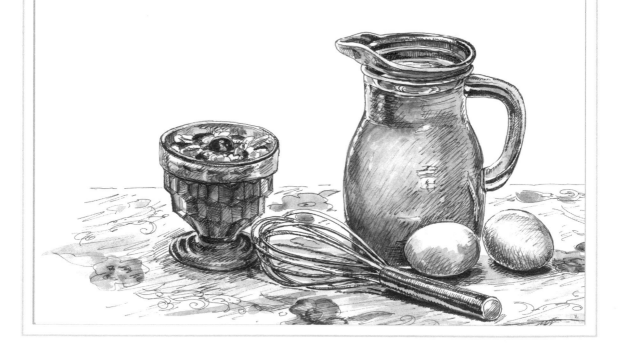

Breakfast Sweet Potatoes

ingredients

3 medium sweet potatoes

1 to 2 tablespoons bacon drippings, olive oil, or butter

Cook the sweet potatoes until tender by either boiling or baking. Peel the cooked sweet potatoes and slice thinly. Heat a skillet with the drippings. When the skillet is hot drop in the sliced sweet potatoes and cook over medium heat until the edges are crisp.

MAKES 4 SERVINGS

This dish is traditionally cooked in a large black skillet and is delicious with grits, bacon or sausage, and eggs.

Spiced Breakfast Chips

ingredients

2 medium sweet potatoes

5 tablespoons butter or margarine

1 teaspoon cinnamon or more
   to taste

2 tablespoons confectioners' sugar

Wash, peel, and very thinly slice the sweet potatoes. Melt the butter in a skillet and sauté the sweet potatoes over high heat, stirring frequently. Transfer the sweet potatoes from the skillet onto paper towels. Blot up the excess butter.

Mix the cinnamon and confectioners' sugar together in a small bowl. Sift onto both sides of the chips.

Brunch Sweet Potatoes and Eggs

ingredients

1 cup shredded sweet potato

5 eggs

5 scallions, finely chopped

½ cup low fat cottage cheese

1 cup finely grated Swiss cheese

1 tablespoon Worcestershire sauce

1 tablespoon finely chopped fresh
  parsley

Salt and freshly ground white
  pepper to taste

Nonstick vegetable spray

½ cup chopped cooked ham
  or bacon

Cook the sweet potato in a microwave on high setting for 3 to 4 minutes or until limp. Beat the eggs in a large bowl. Add the sweet potato. Fold in the chopped scallions, cottage cheese, Swiss cheese, Worcestershire sauce, and parsley. Season with salt and freshly ground white pepper, remembering that either ham or bacon will be added.

Spray a 10-inch glass pie dish or quiche dish with nonstick vegetable spray. Pour mixture into the dish, cover, and refrigerate overnight.

Preheat the oven to 350°. Remove the dish and sprinkle with ham or bacon. Bake for about 35 minutes or until done.

MAKES 6 TO 8 SERVINGS

This is a great dish to serve as you would a quiche for brunch or supper with a tossed salad or cup of hot soup. It may be altered by substituting cilantro for the parsley and 1 teaspoon of hot sauce for the Worcestershire for a spicier version.

Coffee Cake Surprise

ingredients

½ cup shortening

1½ cups sugar

1 egg

3 cups all-purpose flour

2 teaspoons baking powder

1 cup milk

2 sweet potatoes

2 tablespoons sugar

2 teaspoons cinnamon

Preheat the oven to 375° and grease a 9x13-inch baking pan.. Cream together the shortening and sugar in a large mixing bowl. Add the egg and beat well. Sift together the flour and baking powder in a separate bowl. Add the dry ingredients to the creamed mixture alternately with the milk, beating well after each addition (begin and end with dry ingredients). Spread the batter into the baking pan. Meanwhile, peel and thinly slice the sweet potatoes. Arrange on top of the batter. Combine the sugar and cinnamon, and sprinkle over the sweet potatoes. Bake for 40 to 45 minutes. Serve warm.

MAKES 12 SERVINGS

—*Sweet Potato Council of the U.S., Inc.*

Bacon and Orange Sweet Potatoes

ingredients

4 medium sweet potatoes

1 tablespoon maple syrup

¼ cup orange juice concentrate

⅛ teaspoon orange zest

1½ teaspoons chopped fresh thyme

½ pound lean bacon

Preheat the oven to 350°. Wash and peel the sweet potatoes, then julienne in a food processor. Place the sweet potatoes in a microwave proof dish, cover, and microwave on high for 4 minutes. In a glass baking dish toss the sweet potatoes with the maple syrup, orange juice, zest, and fresh thyme. Spray with a nonstick spray. Bake for 20 minutes.

Cook the bacon in the microwave until crisp. Crumble on top of the orange sweet potatoes and serve hot.

MAKES 6 SERVINGS

This is an excellent dish for a brunch. Serve with a crisp green salad and a bread.

Sweet Potato Grits

ingredients

2 cups sweet potatoes, drained

4 cups water

1 cup plain grits

1 clove garlic, peeled and crushed

1 teaspoon salt

½ cup margarine

1 tablespoon Worcestershire sauce

4 egg whites

Preheat the oven to 350° and spray a soufflé dish with nonstick spray. Purée the sweet potatoes in a blender. Bring the water to boil in a heavy saucepan and add the grits, crushed garlic, and salt. Reduce the heat, stir, and cover. Cook over low heat for about 15 minutes, stirring frequently, until the grits are thick.

Add the margarine, puréed sweet potatoes, and Worcestershire sauce. Beat the egg whites in a large bowl until stiff. Fold the egg whites into the sweet potato-grits mixture. Pour the mixture into the prepared dish. Bake for about 35 minutes.

MAKES 4 TO 6 SERVINGS

This brightly colored dish is great for a brunch. Using only the egg whites and margarine makes it a low fat dish. It is best served immediately after baking as it has soufflé properties. It also can be altered and made the day before serving, except for baking, by using whole eggs.

Sweet Potato
main dishes

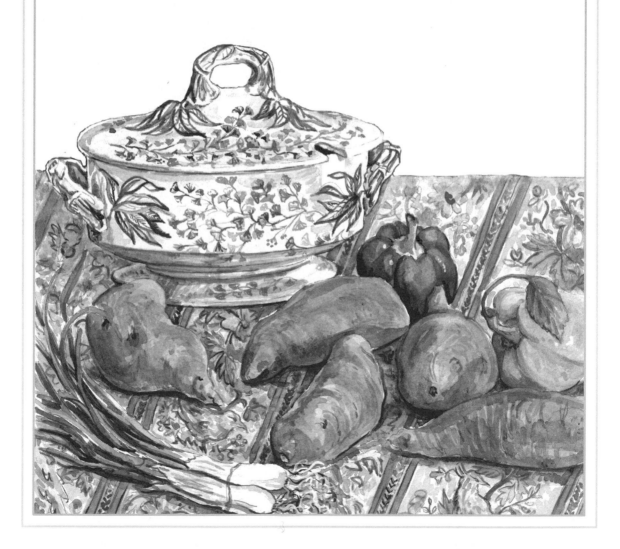

Three Vegetable Stew

ingredients

1 tablespoon olive oil

1 red onion, chopped

2 cloves garlic, minced

6 ounces fresh kale

5 cups stock (vegetable, chicken, or beef)

3 sweet potatoes, peeled and diced

1 teaspoon dry mustard

½ teaspoon grated ginger

2 yellow summer squash, diced

2 ripe tomatoes, diced

2 tablespoons soy sauce

Pepper to taste

1 cup cooked brown rice

Grated Cheddar cheese for topping

Heat the oil in a stock pot and sauté the onion and garlic for about 10 minutes. Wash the kale and remove the hard rib in center. Cut into small pieces. Add to the stock pot with the stock. Add the sweet potatoes and cook about 20 minutes until tender.

Remove the solids and purée in a food processor. Add back to the stock pot. Add the mustard and ginger, stirring well. Cook slowly on medium heat for about 5 minutes. Add the squash and tomatoes, cooking slowly about 15 minutes longer. Add the soy sauce and pepper. Let the stew stand for at least 1 hour before serving.

Serve hot over rice. Top with grated cheese.

MAKES 6 SERVINGS

Chicken Pie with Sweet Potato Crust

ingredients

3 cups diced cooked chicken

1 cup sliced cooked carrots

6 small white onions, quartered
   and cooked

1 tablespoon chopped fresh parsley

3 tablespoons all-purpose flour

1 cup milk

1 cup chicken broth

Salt and pepper to taste

Sweet Potato Crust

2 cups all-purpose flour

1 teaspoon baking powder

½ teaspoon salt

⅓ cup shortening

1 cup cold mashed sweet potatoes

1 egg, well beaten

Preheat the oven to 350°. Layer the chicken, carrots, onion, and parsley in a greased 2½-quart casserole dish. Combine the flour and a small amount of milk in a saucepan, blending until smooth. Gradually stir in the remaining milk and chicken broth. Place over low heat and cook until thickened, stirring constantly. Add salt and pepper. Pour the sauce over the chicken and vegetables in the casserole dish. Cover the mixture with Sweet Potato Crust. Bake for about 45 minutes.

To make the Crust

Combine the flour, baking powder, and salt in a large bowl. Cut in the shortening until the mixture resembles coarse crumbs. Add the sweet potato and egg, blending well. Roll the dough out on a lightly floured surface to ¼-inch thickness.

MAKES 6 TO 8 SERVINGS

Shepherd's Pie

ingredients

3 medium sweet potatoes, steamed,
    peeled, and mashed

1 pound ground beef or turkey

6 tablespoons unsalted butter

1 medium onion, finely chopped

2 cloves garlic, crushed

1 tablespoon chopped fresh thyme

1 cup chicken or beef stock

2 cups chopped tomatoes

1 cup thinly sliced shitaki
    mushrooms

1 tablespoon flour or cornstarch
    for thickening water

Salt and pepper

Worcestershire sauce

1 egg yolk

Preheat the oven to 350° and grease a glass baking dish.

Use a pat of the butter in the bottom of a skillet to brown the chopped onion and mushrooms. Add the ground meat and cook until lightly browned. Remove any fat. Season to taste with salt, pepper, and a little Worcestershire sauce. Remove the meat mixture to the glass baking dish. Mix the flour with a little water to make a paste to add to the cooked meat liquid to thicken. Whisk well and add to casserole dish, blending well.

Mix salt, egg yolk, and remaining butter into the mashed sweet potatoes. Spoon into a pastry bag with a star point. Pipe the sweet potato mixture over the casserole.

Bake for 25 to 30 minutes until lightly browned.

SERVES 4 TO 5 FOR A MAIN COURSE AND 6 TO 8 FOR SIDE DISH

For a tasty variation, try adding grated cheddar or parmesan cheese to the sweet potato topping.

Vegetarian Shepherd's Pie

ingredients

2 tablespoons olive oil

2 medium onions, thinly sliced

2 cloves garlic, crushed

1 tablespoon curry powder

5 cups chopped tomatoes

3 cups chopped eggplant

3 cups chopped broccoli

2 medium parsnips, scraped
  and sliced

2 medium carrots, scraped
  and sliced

4 medium sweet potatoes, steamed,
  peeled, and mashed

6 tablespoons butter

Salt and pepper to taste

Hot sauce to taste

Preheat the oven to 350° and grease a glass casserole dish.

Heat the oil in a skillet, and add the onions and garlic, stirring until onions are soft. Add the curry powder, and mix well. Add the tomatoes, eggplant, broccoli, parsnips, and carrots. Simmer uncovered until vegetables are tender, about 10 minutes. Season with the salt, pepper, and hot sauce. Cool. Spoon the vegetable mixture into the casserole dish. Spread with the mashed sweet potatoes and butter. Bake for 30 minutes until lightly browned.

SERVES 4 TO 5 FOR A MAIN COURSE AND 6 TO 8 FOR SIDE DISH

Tasty Turnovers

ingredients

1 8-ounce package refrigerated crescent rolls

3 cups cubed cooked turkey or chicken

1¼ cups chopped cooked sweet potatoes

1 onion, finely chopped

1 10-ounce package chopped spinach

½ cup jellied cranberry sauce

2 tablespoons turkey or chicken broth

Preheat the oven to 375° and spray a baking sheet with vegetable spray. Working on a lightly floured surface, separate the crescent rolls into four rectangles. Roll each rectangle until it measures 7x7 inches. Mix together the meat, sweet potato, onion, spinach, cranberry sauce, and broth in a medium bowl. Spoon ¼ of the mixture onto half of each rectangle, leaving a ¼-inch border. Lightly brush the edges of the dough with water and fold over, forming triangles. Press the edges with a fork to seal. Poke the tops lightly with a fork to allow steam to escape. Place the turnovers on the baking sheet. Bake for 15 minutes or until lightly browned.

MAKES 4 SERVINGS

—*Sweet Potato Council of the U.S., Inc.*

Sunday Night Supper Casserole

ingredients

2 medium sweet potatoes

2 tablespoons butter

2 tablespoons milk

Kosher salt

Freshly ground white pepper

8 large slices turkey or ham

1 cup Béchamel sauce (optional)

½ cup chopped walnuts or almonds

Wash the sweet potatoes and boil in water about 30 minutes until tender. Drain, cool, and peel. Place in a food processor and purée, adding the butter, milk, salt, and white pepper. Spray an oven-proof serving dish with vegetable spray. Cover the bottom of the dish with four stacks of meat, each having two slices. Spread Béchamel sauce on each stack and top with a layer of puréed sweet potato mixture. If desired, sprinkle with chopped walnuts or almonds. Bake for 30 minutes.

MAKES 4 SERVINGS

Sunday night dinners were always leftovers, soup, "whatever you can find in the refrigerator," and later, as my children got older, Domino's pizza. This is a super way to use leftover ham, pork tenderloin, turkey, or chicken slices to make a great supper.

Our Favorite Pork and Sweet Potato Dinner

ingredients

8 pork chops, ½-inch thick

⅓ cup all-purpose flour

¼ cup butter or margarine

Salt and pepper to taste

2 cups apple juice, divided

2 pounds small red potatoes

1 pound small whole onions, peeled

4 carrots, peeled and cut into
  3-inch pieces

4 medium sweet potatoes, peeled
  and cut into 1-inch pieces

6 cups shredded cabbage

Preheat the oven to 350°. Coat the pork chops in flour, reserving the excess flour. Melt the butter over medium-high heat in a large Dutch oven. Brown the chops on both sides, seasoning with salt and pepper. Remove and set aside. Stir the reserved flour into the drippings in the pan. Cook and stir until a paste forms. Gradually whisk in 1½ cups apple juice, blending until smooth. Return the chops to Dutch oven and cover. Bake for 30 minutes.

Add the potatoes, onions, carrots, sweet potatoes, and remaining apple juice. Cover and bake for 30 minutes longer.

Top with the cabbage, cover, and bake for 1 hour or until the pork chops are tender, basting occasionally with juices.

MAKES 8 SERVINGS

—*Sweet Potato Council of the U.S., Inc.*

Just Right Casserole

ingredients

1 pound link sausage (pork or turkey)

¼ cup water

4 cooked sweet potatoes, peeled and sliced

1 cup sliced apples

¼ cup firmly packed brown sugar

1 teaspoon salt

3 tablespoons butter or margarine, sliced

Preheat the oven to 375° and butter a baking dish. Simmer the sausage in the water in a skillet for 10 minutes. Do not pierce. Drain.

Arrange one-third of the potatoes in the baking dish. Cover with half the apples. Sprinkle with half the sugar, salt, and butter. Repeat. End with the potatoes. Cover and bake for 30 minutes.

Uncover and arrange the sausage on top. Continue baking uncovered for about 15 minutes or until the apples are tender and the potatoes are lightly browned. Add water if necessary.

MAKES 4 TO 6 SERVINGS

—*Sweet Potato Council of the U.S., Inc.*

Sweet Potatoes and Ham L'Orange

ingredients

3 tablespoons vegetable oil

1 tablespoon butter or margarine

1 16-ounce can small onions, drained

1 pound sweet potatoes, peeled and cubed

1 pound cooked ham, cut into ¼-inch cubes

3 tablespoons all-purpose flour

3 cups chicken broth

¾ cup orange juice

1 teaspoon grated orange peel

½ teaspoon ground pepper

2 cups broccoli florets

Heat the oil and butter over medium heat in a 5-quart Dutch oven. Add the onions and sauté, stirring occasionally, for 8 minutes or until golden.

Transfer to a large plate. Add the sweet potatoes to the Dutch oven and sauté for 5 minutes or until lightly browned. Transfer to the plate. Add ham and sauté for 5 minutes or until lightly browned. Transfer to a separate plate. Whisk the flour into the drippings in the Dutch oven and cook over medium heat, stirring constantly, for 2 minutes. Gradually add the chicken broth and orange juice and cook, stirring constantly, for 3 to 5 minutes or until slightly thickened. Stir in the orange peel and pepper.

Return the sweet potatoes to the Dutch oven, bring to a boil, and cook over medium heat for 10 minutes or until almost tender. Add the ham, onions, and broccoli. Return to a boil, cover, and cook for 10 minutes or until all the vegetables are tender.

MAKES 4 TO 6 SERVINGS

—*Sweet Potato Council of the U.S., Inc.*

Highlands Apple, Sausage, and Sweet Potato Bake

ingredients

1 pound hot country link sausage or patties

1 can sweet potatoes

2 apples

3 tablespoons lemon juice

1 tablespoon all-purpose flour or cornstarch

1 can vegetable, chicken, or beef broth

½ cup sugar

Cook the sausage links in a skillet on medium heat until done. If using sausage patties, you may cook in a microwave according to the package directions. Either way, wipe away as much grease with a paper towel as possible. Drain the sweet potatoes and slice. Peel, core, and slice the apples. Pour lemon juice over the apple slices. Spray a 1-quart casserole dish with vegetable spray. Layer the sausage, sweet potatoes, and apples with lemon juice in the casserole dish.

Preheat the oven to 350°. Place the flour or cornstarch in a saucepan, blending in the broth with a whisk. Add the sugar. Simmer until thickened. Pour over the sweet potatoes, apples, and sausage. Bake for about 15 to 20 minutes.

MAKES 4 TO 6 SERVINGS

This makes a great winter supper dish with a green salad, crunchy coleslaw, corn bread, and dessert.

Sweet Potato Pork Stir Fry

ingredients

2 medium sweet potatoes

1¼ pound pork tenderloin

2 tablespoons vegetable oil

½ teaspoon salt

½ cup water

⅓ cup chopped green onions

2 tablespoons raisins

1½ teaspoons cornstarch

2 tablespoons cooking wine

2 cups thinly sliced tart apples

Wash and peel the sweet potatoes. Cut into strips like French fries. Cut the pork diagonally into slices ¼-inch thick. Stir fry the pork in hot oil in a wok or heavy skillet until done. Remove from the wok and season with salt. Add the sweet potatoes and water. Cover and cook for 5 to 7 minutes, stirring occasionally. Add the pork, onions, and raisins. Combine the cornstarch and wine in a cup to make a paste. Stir into the sweet potato and pork mixture. Cook and stir until the sauce is thickened. Fold in the apple slices. Serve immediately.

MAKES 4 TO 6 SERVINGS

Baked Pineapple, Sausage, and Sweet Potatoes

ingredients

4 large sweet potatoes

1 pound sausage patties

2 strips bacon, minced

8 pineapple slices

¼ cup pineapple juice

¼ cup firmly packed brown sugar

Preheat the oven to 350° and spray a casserole dish with vegetable spray. Boil the sweet potatoes in salted water in a large pot until tender. Drain, cool, peel, and slice. Cook the sausage patties and bacon in a skillet. Drain and pat the grease off. Place a layer of sweet potatoes in the bottom of the casserole. Add the sausage and bacon mixture next, followed with the pineapple slices. Top with the remaining sweet potatoes, pouring pineapple juice over the sweet potatoes. Sprinkle with the brown sugar. Bake for 45 minutes in the center of the oven.

MAKES 4 TO 6 SERVINGS

Southwestern Vegetable One Dish Meal

ingredients

1 can sweet potatoes, drained

2 tablespoons olive oil

1 onion, finely chopped

4 cloves garlic

2 tomatoes, chopped

1 cup frozen broccoli

1 cup frozen peas

⅓ cup water

Salt and pepper to taste

Topping

1 egg

1 tablespoon sugar

½ cup milk

½ cup cornmeal

½ cup self-rising flour

¼ cup canned corn

1 teaspoon chopped and seeded
  jalapeño

2 tablespoons chopped pimento

Preheat the oven to 400° and spray a 2-quart glass casserole dish with vegetable spray. Cut the drained sweet potatoes into slices. Heat the oil in a large skillet and sauté the onion and garlic. Add the sweet potatoes, tomatoes, broccoli, peas, and water. Cover and simmer for about 8 minutes on low heat. Season with salt and pepper. Pour the vegetable mixture into the casserole dish.

To make the Topping

Beat the egg with the sugar in the bowl of an electric mixer on medium speed, adding the milk. Combine the cornmeal and flour in a separate bowl. Add to the egg mixture. Fold in the corn, jalapeño, and pimento.

Spread over the vegetables and bake for 20 minutes or until a wooden toothpick comes out clean.

MAKES 6 SERVINGS

Highlands Trout and Sweet Potatoes

ingredients

Béchamel Sauce

2 tablespoons butter

1½ tablespoons all-purpose flour

1 cup milk

1 onion studded with cloves

1 bay leaf

Saffron-Fennel Sauce

¼ cup white wine

¼ cup fish stock

2 white peppercorns

¼ teaspoon saffron

4 sprigs blanched fennel sprigs

1 teaspoon finely chopped onion

Trout

1 medium sweet potato

2 tablespoons lemon juice

4 rainbow trout fillets

1 egg, beaten

1 tablespoon butter

Salt and freshly ground white
  pepper to taste

Prepare the Béchamel as follows and set aside

Melt the butter in a small saucepan, adding the flour and blending well to make a white roux. Slowly stir in the milk. Add the clove-studded onion and a bay leaf. Cook and stir very slowly with a wire whisk until smooth and thick. Strain the sauce.

To make the Saffron-Fennel Sauce

Combine the white wine, fish stock, peppercorns, saffron, fennel, and onion in a saucepan and cook slowly over medium heat for about 5 minutes, stirring constantly. Strain the sauce and add the Béchamel sauce made earlier.

The sauces can be prepared the day before and heated in a double boiler when ready to serve.

To make the Trout

Scrub and peel the sweet potato. Shred in a food processor. Combine the shredded sweet potato with the lemon juice, cover, and microwave for 2 minutes or until limp. Drain the lemon juice off and pour it over the trout fillets.

Brush the trout with the egg. Melt the butter in a skillet. Add the trout, cover with shredded sweet potato, and sauté until done. Turn once. Season with salt and pepper.

To serve, make a bed of the saffron-fennel sauce and top with the trout and sweet potatoes. Garnish with fennel sprigs.

The sauce that complements the trout is a white wine fish sauce made with a basic Béchamel flavored with saffron and fennel.

The above recipe can be changed in numerous ways. Substitute salmon fillets for the rainbow trout. Change the sauce and use tarragon in place of the saffron and fennel for either rainbow trout or salmon.

Sausage Sweet Potato Casserole

ingredients

1 pound lean sausage meat

1½ cups thinly sliced apples

¼ cup firmly packed brown sugar

2 cups cooked sweet potatoes,

¼ teaspoon salt

½ cup milk

Preheat the oven to 350°. Place the sausage in a baking dish. Arrange the apple slices on top of the sausage. Sprinkle with brown sugar. Mash the sweet potatoes, add salt and milk, and beat until light and fluffy. Place the sweet potato mixture on the apple slices. Bake for 1 hour. Serve very hot.

MAKES 4 TO 6 SERVINGS

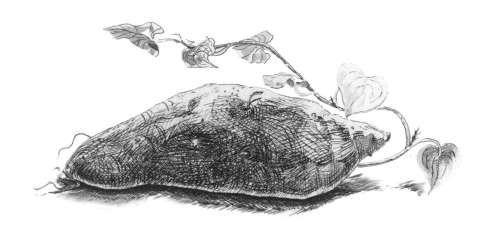

Sweet Potato Dumplings

ingredients

3 medium sweet potatoes

1 teaspoon salt

¼ teaspoon freshly ground nutmeg

⅛ teaspoon cayenne pepper

2 eggs

½ cup all-purpose flour

Chicken or vegetable stock (see pages 15–17)

Wash the sweet potatoes and boil in water about 30 minutes until tender. Drain, cool, and peel. Place in a food processor and purée. Add the salt, nutmeg, cayenne pepper, and eggs, and mix until smooth. Add the flour and blend well. Dust hands with flour and roll a teaspoonful of dough into dumplings. Drop into boiling chicken stock and cook 5 minutes. Reduce the heat and simmer for 5 minutes more.

MAKES 6 SERVINGS

Sweet Potatoes Stewed

ingredients

4 medium sweet potatoes, peeled

¼ pound country ham

8 pieces chicken

¼ teaspoon marjoram

¼ teaspoon thyme

¼ teaspoon basil

Salt and pepper to taste

1 cup chicken broth

1 tablespoon butter

2 tablespoons all-purpose flour

Preheat the oven to 350°. Place the sweet potatoes in the bottom of a Dutch oven. Add the ham, chicken pieces, marjoram, thyme, basil, salt, pepper. Pour in the chicken broth, cover, and bake for 1 hour until chicken and potatoes are tender.

Remove the chicken and potatoes from the pan and place in a serving dish. Keep warm. Skim off as much fat as possible from the cooking liquid. To thicken the gravy, in a saucepan melt the butter and stir in the flour. Blend in the cooking liquid. Bring to boil, reduce the heat, and simmer 10 minutes. Adjust the seasonings.

Pour the gravy over the chicken and potatoes to serve.

This flavorful stew is a more genteel version of "Possum & Sweet Potatoes," a favorite dish of the Old South.

Sausage Stuffing

ingredients

1 pound ground pork sausage

1 large onion, chopped

½ cup chopped celery

½ cup chopped green bell pepper

3 cups mashed cooked sweet
   potatoes

1 teaspoon grated orange peel

¼ cup finely chopped parsley

1 cup chicken broth

½ cup orange juice

2 eggs, beaten

2 8-ounce packages corn bread
   stuffing mix

Preheat the oven to 350° and spray a large casserole dish with vegetable spray. Brown the sausage in a skillet. Drain. Sauté the onion, celery, and green pepper in the same skillet until tender. Combine the sausage, vegetables, sweet potatoes, orange peel, and parsley in a large bowl. Add the chicken broth, orange juice, and eggs, blending well. Combine with the stuffing mix. Transfer the stuffing mix to the prepared dish. Bake for 1 hour.

MAKES 10 TO 12 SERVINGS

WILL STUFF A 16- TO 20-POUND TURKEY

San Francisco Sweet Potato Stir Fry

ingredients

¼ cup hoisin sauce

¼ cup soy sauce

2 tablespoons balsamic vinegar

2 teaspoons brown sugar

1 teaspoon sesame oil

¼ teaspoon garlic powder

¼ teaspoon black pepper

1 pound boneless chicken breast
or pork cutlets

2 tablespoons cooking oil

1 large sweet potato, peeled and
sliced

1 large onion, sliced

1 large carrot, thinly sliced

½ pound snow peas

½ pound asparagus, sliced on bias

2 teaspoons cornstarch

1 cup chopped Chinese cabbage

Hot cooked rice

For the marinade, in a medium bowl combine the hoisin sauce, soy sauce, vinegar, brown sugar, sesame oil, garlic powder, and pepper. Cut the meat into bite-size strips. Add the chicken or pork to the marinade. Toss to coat; cover and refrigerate for 1 to 24 hours.

Heat 1 tablespoon of the cooking oil in a wok or skillet over medium-high heat. Add the sweet potato, onion, carrot, snow peas, and asparagus. Stir fry for 4 to 5 minutes or until tender crisp. Remove the vegetables from the wok or skillet. Drain the meat well, reserving the marinade. Stir the cornstarch into the marinade and set aside. Heat the remaining cooking oil in the wok or skillet. Add the meat and stir fry for 3 minutes or until no pink remains. Remove from the wok. Add the marinade to the wok. Cook and stir over medium heat until thick and bubbly. Return the meat and vegetables to the wok. Add the cabbage and heat through. Serve over hot cooked rice.

MAKES 4 SERVINGS

—*Sweet Potato Council of the U.S., Inc.*

Chicken Oriental Sweet Potatoes

ingredients

5 medium sweet potatoes

1 fryer chicken, cut into parts

1 cup soy sauce

3 tablespoons brown sugar

¼ cup dry sherry

1 teaspoon ground ginger

3 cloves garlic, crushed

Hot cooked rice

Chopped green onion

Wash and peel the sweet potatoes. Cut each sweet potato into four pieces lengthwise. Arrange the sweet potato pieces and chicken in a glass baking dish. Combine the soy sauce, brown sugar, sherry, ginger, and garlic in a medium bowl, mixing well. Pour over the sweet potatoes and chicken. Cover and marinate in the refrigerator for at least 2 hours, turning once. Preheat the oven to 350°. Bake for 25 minutes.

Turn the chicken and sweet potatoes and baste. Bake 20 minutes longer or until the chicken is done.

Arrange the chicken and sweet potatoes over hot cooked rice and sprinkle with chopped green onions.

MAKES 6 TO 8 SERVINGS

Savory and Sweet Kabobs

ingredients

¼ teaspoon salt

½ teaspoon dried oregano

¼ teaspoon ginger

¼ teaspoon allspice

2 tablespoons finely chopped scallions

½ teaspoon black pepper

1 clove garlic, minced

½ teaspoon Worcestershire sauce

1 pound beef top round, cut into ¼-inch cubes

2 medium sweet potatoes, peeled

1 large red bell pepper, seeded

1 medium zucchini, thickly sliced

Combine all of the seasonings in a large self-sealing plastic food storage bag. Add the beef, seal, and shake gently to coat the beef. Refrigerate for 2 hours.

Cut the sweet potatoes into quarters and cook in boiling water for 4 minutes or until almost tender. Drain well and rinse in cold water. Cut the pepper into large strips. Thread the beef on four 10-inch metal skewers, alternating with the sweet potato, red pepper, and zucchini. Cook on a grill for 10 minutes, turning after 5 minutes (the skewers should be about 6 inches above the coals). The kabobs may also be arranged on a foil-lined broiler pan. Broil for 8 minutes, turning once.

MAKES 4 SERVINGS

—*Sweet Potato Council of the U.S., Inc.*

Sweet and Perfect Pork with Raisin Sauce

ingredients

3 boneless pork loin butterfly
   chops, ½-inch thick

1 tablespoon butter

Salt to taste

⅔ cup orange juice

2 tablespoons raisins

½ teaspoon dry mustard

⅛ teaspoon allspice

3 medium sweet potatoes, cooked
   and peeled

Using a meat mallet, pound each pork loin butterfly chop to about ¼-inch thick. Melt the butter in a 12-inch skillet over medium high heat, and cook the pork for 5 minutes or until tender, browned, and cooked through. Turn only once. Sprinkle with salt. Remove the pork chops to a warm platter and keep warm.

Stir the orange juice, raisins, dry mustard, and allspice into the remaining drippings, stirring to loosen the bits from the skillet. Cook, stirring constantly, until the sauce boils and thickens slightly.

Slice the sweet potatoes into ½-inch thick pieces and add to the skillet. Heat through. Spoon the potatoes onto the platter with the pork chops. Pour the sauce over the chops and sweet potatoes.

MAKES 2 SERVINGS

—*Sweet Potato Council of the U.S., Inc.*

Carrot and Sweet Potato Tzimmes

ingredients

8 pitted prunes

¼ cup boiling water

1 onion, thinly sliced

2 carrots, thinly sliced

2 apples, peeled and sliced

1 cup chicken broth

1 29-ounce can sweet potatoes, drained

⅔ cup orange juice

2 tablespoons lemon juice

1 tablespoon honey

1 teaspoon orange zest

¼ teaspoon freshly grated nutmeg

¼ teaspoon cinnamon

Salt, if needed

Preheat the oven to 350°. Spray a 9x13-inch oven-proof baking dish with nonstick spray. Soak the prunes in the hot water for about 15 minutes.

Cut the prunes in half.

Cook the onion, carrots, and apples in a saucepan with the chicken broth for 8 to 10 minutes over medium high heat. Combine all the ingredients in the saucepan and pour into the prepared baking dish. Cover and cook for 1 hour.

MAKES 8 SERVINGS

Chinese Steamed Beef with Sweet Potatoes

ingredients

1½ tablespoons soy sauce

1 tablespoon brown bean sauce

1 teaspoon sugar

1 tablespoon sherry

1 teaspoon sesame oil

1 teaspoon chopped ginger

½ teaspoon water

1 pound beef tenderloin, sliced very thin against grain

2 cups cooked, mashed sweet potatoes

Salt to taste

2 tablespoons butter

Combine the soy sauce, brown bean sauce, sugar, sherry, sesame oil, chopped ginger, and water in a shallow dish, and mix well. Add the beef, cover, and refrigerate for several hours.

Remove the meat from the marinade. Steam the beef in a steamer over boiling water for 30 to 45 minutes or until the beef is tender and soft.

In a large serving dish mix the sweet potatoes with salt and butter. Place the beef on top of the sweet potatoes.

MAKES 6 TO 8 SERVINGS

Sweet Potato
side dishes

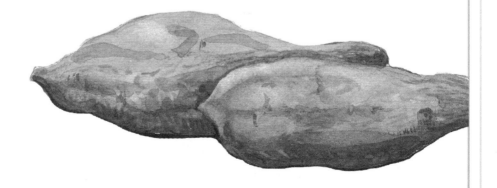

Tropical Sweet Potatoes Gratin

ingredients

6 medium sweet potatoes

¾ cup heavy cream

¼ cup brown sugar plus two
   tablespoons, divided

1 teaspoon orange zest

½ cup orange juice

1 teaspoon ground coriander

1 teaspoon salt

½ teaspoon ground ginger

2 tablespoons butter or margarine,
   melted

Preheat the oven to 350° and spray a gratin dish with vegetable spray. Wash and peel the sweet potatoes. Julienne the sweet potatoes in a food processor. Bring the heavy cream, sweet potatoes, ¼ cup brown sugar, orange zest, orange juice, coriander, salt, and ginger just to a boil in a large saucepan, stirring constantly.

Spoon the mixture into the gratin dish and cover with aluminum foil. Bake for 1 hour. Remove the cover. Drizzle with melted butter, sprinkle the remaining brown sugar over the top, and bake for 15 minutes longer.

Pineapple Sweet Potato Kabobs

ingredients

4 medium sweet potatoes
1 21-ounce can pineapple chunks,
    drained

Scrub the sweet potatoes. Cover the sweet potatoes with hot water in a large pot and boil for 10 to 15 minutes until partially cooked. Drain and cool. Peel and cut into thick cubes. Alternate sweet potato chunks with pineapple chunks on soaked bamboo skewers. Spray with nonstick butter spray. Grill over very hot coals until browned. Spray often with the butter spray while grilling.

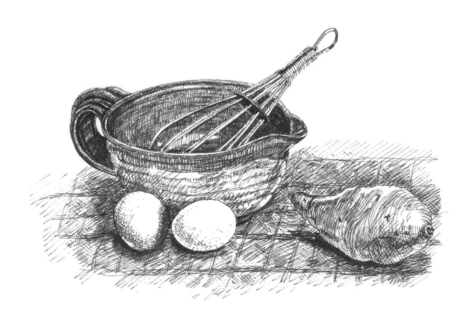

Iberian Sweet Potatoes

ingredients

3 medium sweet potatoes

3 tablespoons olive oil

1 Vidalia or sweet onion, chopped

2 bay leaves

2 tablespoons chopped fresh chives

¼ teaspoon salt

Lemon pepper to taste

1½ cups sherry

Scrub the sweet potatoes. Cover the sweet potatoes in hot water in a large pot and boil for 10 to 15 minutes until partially cooked. Drain and cool. Peel and cut into thick cubes. Heat the olive oil in a large skillet and sauté the onion until tender. Add the sweet potatoes, bay leaves, chives, salt, lemon pepper, and sherry. Bring just to a boil. Reduce the heat, cover, and cook on low heat for about 35 to 40 minutes until the sweet potatoes are done. Remove the bay leaves and serve immediately.

MAKES 6 TO 8 SERVINGS

Pineapple Sweet Potato Bake

ingredients

6 medium sweet potatoes

¼ cup margarine

2 eggs

2 teaspoons orange zest

¼ teaspoon salt

1 8-ounce can pineapple chunks,
drained

Preheat the oven to 325° and spray a glass baking dish with vegetable spray. Scrub the sweet potatoes. Cook the sweet potatoes in a large pot of boiling water for 30 minutes or until tender. Drain, cool, and peel. Purée the sweet potatoes in a food processor, and add the margarine. Add the eggs, orange zest, and salt. Pulse the food processor until thoroughly blended. Stir in the pineapple chunks. Pour the sweet potato mixture into the baking dish and spread evenly. Cover and bake for 45 minutes.

MAKES 6 TO 8 SERVINGS

Summer Casserole

ingredients

1 29-ounce can sweet potatoes, drained

1 8¼-ounce can pineapple chunks

1 8-ounce package cream cheese

½ cup papaya juice

¼ teaspoon freshly grated nutmeg

½ cup Macadamia nuts (optional)

Preheat the oven to 350°, and spray a glass baking dish with nonstick spray. Slice the sweet potatoes. Drain the pineapple, reserving the juice. Add enough water to the juice to measure ½ cup. Combine the cream cheese, papaya juice, and pineapple juice in a saucepan. Stir over low heat until creamy. Place the drained sweet potato slices, Macadamia nuts, and pineapple chunks in the bottom of the casserole. Sprinkle with freshly grated nutmeg. Spoon the hot cream cheese mixture over the sweet potato pineapple mixture. Bake about 15 minutes.

MAKES 6 SERVINGS

Butternut Squash Purée

ingredients

2 butternut squash

1 29-ounce can sweet potatoes, drained

½ cup margarine

½ cup half and half

½ teaspoon salt

½ teaspoon freshly grated nutmeg

¼ cup firmly packed brown sugar

Preheat the oven to 350°, and spray a glass baking dish with nonstick spray. Peel the squash, remove the seeds and strings, and slice. Place in a microwave-safe dish with 2 tablespoons of water, cover, and cook on high for 3 to 5 minutes until tender. Drain off the water. Purée the sweet potatoes and butternut squash in a food processor. Add the margarine, half and half, salt, nutmeg, and brown sugar, and blend well. Pour the purée into the prepared dish and bake for 20 minutes.

MAKES 8 SERVINGS

Sherried Apples and Sweet Potatoes

ingredients

3 medium sweet potatoes

3 Granny Smith apples

¼ cup freshly squeezed lemon juice

2 tablespoons brown sugar

¼ teaspoon freshly grated nutmeg

⅓ cup sherry

Scrub the sweet potatoes and boil for about 30 minutes until tender. Drain, peel, and cube the sweet potatoes. While the sweet potatoes are cooking, peel, core, and cube the apples. Dip the apples in lemon juice. Spray a large skillet with vegetable spray and cook the apples over medium heat until soft. Stir in the brown sugar, lemon juice, nutmeg, and sherry. Continue stirring and cook about 5 minutes more. Add the sweet potatoes and cook until hot. Serve immediately.

MAKES 6 SERVINGS

New England Candied Sweet Potatoes

ingredients

3 medium sweet potatoes

6 tablespoons brandy

¼ cup maple syrup

3 tablespoons freshly squeezed
  lemon juice

Preheat the oven to 350°. Wash and boil the sweet potatoes in water about 30 minutes until tender. Drain, cool, peel, and slice in ½-inch pieces. Spray a shallow baking dish with nonstick spray and place the sweet potatoes slices in a single layer. Sprinkle each slice with the brandy. Drizzle the maple syrup over all the slices. Bake for about 30 minutes. Sprinkle with the lemon juice. Cook 10 minutes more. Finish browning under the broiler for about 3 minutes or until brown.

MAKES 4 TO 6 SERVINGS

Cranberries and Sweet Potatoes

ingredients

1 16-ounce can sweet potatoes,
    drained

½ teaspoon cinnamon

1 16-ounce can whole cranberry
    sauce

Preheat the oven to 350°, and spray a glass baking dish with vegetable spray. Spread the sweet potatoes in the baking dish. Sprinkle with cinnamon. Spread the cranberry sauce over sweet potatoes. Bake for 15 to 20 minutes.

MAKES 6 SERVINGS

Whipped Sweet Potatoes

ingredients

5 medium sweet potatoes

2 tablespoons unsalted butter

1 tablespoon finely chopped
fresh thyme

Kosher salt

Freshly ground white pepper

Preheat the oven to 350°. Scrub the sweet potatoes and spray with nonstick spray. Spray a baking sheet with nonstick spray and place the sweet potatoes on the sheet. Bake for 1 hour and 15 minutes or until tender when speared with a cooking fork.

Take the sweet potatoes out of the oven, cool, peel, and purée. Melt the butter in a saucepan and add the puréed sweet potatoes and the chopped thyme. Season with Kosher salt and freshly ground white pepper.

MAKES 6 TO 8 SERVINGS

Bacon Stuffed Sweet Potatoes

ingredients

6 large sweet potatoes

1 cup low fat sour cream

¼ cup margarine

½ teaspoon salt

1 egg, beaten

Freshly ground white pepper

1 teaspoon sugar

12 bacon slices, cooked and
   crumbled

Paprika

Preheat oven to 400°. Wash the sweet potatoes and spray with nonstick vegetable spray. Place on a baking sheet and bake for about 1 hour or until done throughout.

Cut in half lengthwise and scoop out the pulp, saving the shells. Add the sour cream, margarine, salt, egg, freshly ground white pepper, and sugar to the pulp. Processor purée the mixture in a food processor. Add the crumbled bacon. Fill the potato shells with the mixture and sprinkle paprika on top. Bake for about 8 to 10 minutes or until heated through.

MAKES 10 TO 12 SERVINGS

Cranberry Glazed Sweet Potatoes

ingredients

6 medium sweet potatoes
1 cup whole berry cranberry sauce
½ cup water
¼ cup firmly packed brown sugar
½ teaspoon grated orange peel
1 tablespoon margarine

Preheat the oven to 400°. Scrub the sweet potatoes and spray with vegetable spray. Place on a baking sheet. Bake for about 40 minutes or until soft. Cool, peel, and slice lengthwise.

Arrange the sweet potatoes in a shallow, non-stick vegetable-sprayed baking dish flat side down. Combine cranberry sauce, water, brown sugar, and orange peel in a saucepan and bring to a boil. Reduce the heat and cook for 5 minutes, stirring frequently. Add the margarine and pour the mixture over the sweet potatoes. Reduce the oven temperature to 350° and bake for about 30 minutes, basting frequently.

MAKES 4 TO 6 SERVINGS

Sweet Potato Timbales

ingredients

4 medium sweet potatoes

1 teaspoon finely chopped fresh
   chives

Kosher salt

2 tablespoons half and half

4 egg whites

Crème Fraîche (see page 26)

Pepper Rouille

1 onion, chopped

1 tablespoon olive oil

3 red bell peppers, seeded and
   chopped

1 clove garlic, peeled and crushed

2 cups chopped tomato

1 teaspoon paprika

Preheat the oven to 350°. Wash the sweet potatoes and boil in water about 30 minutes until tender. Spray 8 ramekins with nonstick spray. Drain, cool, peel, and purée the potatoes. Add the chives, a pinch of Kosher salt, and half and half to the sweet potato purée and process again. Beat the egg whites into stiff peaks in a large bowl. Fold the egg whites into the sweet potato purée and divide between the 8 ramekins. Cover the tops with parchment paper or waxed paper. Place the filled ramekins in a baking pan filled with hot water two-thirds up the sides of the ramekins. Bake for 30 minutes or until set. Serve immediately.

Serve with Crème Fraîche spooned on top or a Pepper Rouille.

To make a Pepper Rouille

Heat the olive oil in a skillet and sauté the onion and peppers until limp. Add the crushed garlic, tomato, and paprika. Cover, reduce the heat, and cook for about 5 minutes. Remove from the heat and cool. Purée the pepper mixture in a food processor, and strain. Serve on top of the Sweet Potato Timbales.

Glazed Sweet Potatoes

ingredients

⅓ cup water

1 3-ounce package orange-flavored gelatin

¼ teaspoon cinnamon

Dash salt

2 tablespoons margarine

1 16-ounce can sweet potatoes, drained

Mix together the water, gelatin, cinnamon, and dash of salt in a skillet. Add the margarine. Bring to the boiling point, stirring constantly. Add the sweet potatoes. Reduce the heat, cover, and cook for about 15 minutes until the sweet potatoes are glazed.

MAKES 4 SERVINGS

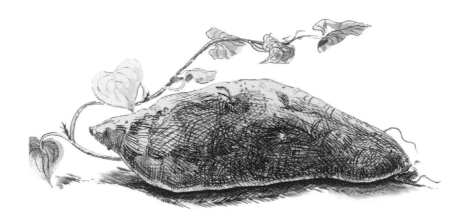

Apple Glazed Sweet Potatoes

ingredients

½ cup apple jelly

Fresh mint, chopped

Dash salt

¼ teaspoon freshly grated nutmeg

1 can sweet potatoes, drained

Melt the jelly in a skillet over low heat. Stir in the chopped mint, salt, nutmeg, and sweet potatoes. Cook over low heat about 5 minutes, turning the sweet potatoes several times until well coated and most of the juice is absorbed.

MAKES 4 TO 6 SERVINGS

Herbed Sweet Potato Bake

ingredients

2 cups mashed cooked sweet
   potatoes
1 8-ounce package cream cheese,
   softened
¼ cup milk
2 eggs
¾ teaspoon basil
¾ teaspoon thyme
½ teaspoon lemon peel
½ teaspoon salt
¼ teaspoon white pepper
¾ cup chopped green onion

Preheat the oven to 350°, and spray a glass baking dish with vegetable spray. Blend the sweet potatoes, cream cheese, milk, eggs, herbs, lemon peel, salt, pepper, and ⅔ cup of the chopped onion together in a large bowl with a mixer at medium speed. Beat until light and fluffy. Spoon the sweet potato mixture into the baking dish. Bake uncovered for 30 to 35 minutes. Sprinkle with the remaining onion.

MAKES 6 TO 8 SERVINGS

Scalloped Sweet Potatoes

ingredients

4 cups sliced raw sweet potatoes

¼ cup margarine, melted, plus
  2 tablespoons

1 medium onion, chopped

1 10½-ounce can cream of
  celery soup

½ teaspoon salt

⅛ teaspoon white pepper

½ cup shredded Cheddar cheese

2 cups herb seasoned stuffing mix

Preheat the oven to 350°, and spray a 2-quart glass baking dish with vegetable spray. Cook the sweet potatoes in a large pot in a small amount of boiling water for 10 minutes or until tender. Drain. Melt 2 tablespoons of margarine in a skillet over medium heat, and sauté the onion until tender, stirring constantly. Stir in the soup, salt, pepper, and cheese. Combine with sweet potatoes.

Spoon the sweet potato mixture into the prepared dish. Combine the stuffing mix and ¼ cup melted margarine in a medium bowl, and spread over the sweet potato mixture. Bake for 20 minutes.

MAKES 6 TO 8 SERVINGS

Highlands Brandied Sweet Potatoes

ingredients

4 medium sweet potatoes

⅔ cup brown sugar

¼ cup water

2 tablespoons butter

½ cup chopped tart apple

¼ cup golden raisins

⅓ cup cognac

Preheat the oven to 350°, and spray a casserole dish with nonstick vegetable spray. Cover the sweet potatoes in water and boil until tender in a large pot. Drain and cool. Peel and slice. Bring the brown sugar, water, butter, and chopped apple to a boil in a saucepan. Add the raisins and stir for 1 minute on low heat. Remove from the heat and add the cognac. Layer the sweet potato slices in the prepared dish. Pour the cognac mixture over the sweet potatoes. Bake uncovered for 30 minutes, basting with the sauce.

MAKES 4 TO 6 SERVINGS

Southern Bourbon Sweet Potatoes

ingredients

5 cups canned sweet potatoes

1 8-ounce can crushed pineapple

2 eggs

5 tablespoons butter, melted

1 cup firmly packed brown sugar

5 tablespoons bourbon

⅓ cup sweetened condensed milk

Topping

½ cup chopped pecans

2 cups Grape Nuts cereal

¼ cup margarine, melted

Preheat the oven to 375°. Spray a 2-quart casserole dish with vegetable spray. Drain the sweet potatoes and crushed pineapple. Combine the sweet potatoes, eggs, butter, brown sugar, bourbon, and condensed milk in a food processor. Pulse to blend until well mixed. Pour the sweet potato mixture into the dish. Add the pineapple and mix gently. This can be made the day before and stored covered in the refrigerator.

To make the Topping

Combine the pecans, Grape Nuts, and margarine in a small bowl. Sprinkle over the casserole. Bake for 20 to 25 minutes.

Garlic Sweet Potatoes

ingredients

2 sweet potatoes

2 tablespoons butter or margarine

1½ tablespoons grated onion

1 clove garlic, mashed

Fresh thyme

3 tablespoons nonfat plain yogurt

¼ teaspoon salt

Pinch white pepper

Preheat the oven to 375°. Place the sweet potatoes on a baking sheet. Bake for 1 hour. Cool and peel. Purée the sweet potatoes in a food processor. Melt the butter in a skillet and sauté the onion and garlic, adding the thyme at the last minute. Add the sautéed mixture, yogurt, salt, and pepper to the puréed sweet potatoes.

This dish can be made a day before serving and reheated in the microwave.

MAKES 4 TO 6 SERVINGS

Anna Sweet Potatoes

ingredients

4 medium sweet potatoes

½ cup butter, melted

Salt and freshly ground white
  pepper to taste

⅓ cup Parmesan cheese

Preheat the oven to 425°. Cut aluminum foil to fit the bottom of a 9-inch cake pan. Rub with butter and set aside. Wash, peel, and slice the sweet potatoes very thinly in round shapes. Wipe the bottom of the cake pan with melted butter. Cover the bottom of pan with sweet potato slices, overlapping each slice. Drizzle a little butter over and sprinkle with salt, pepper, and Parmesan cheese. Continue layering until complete. Press aluminum foil over the top and compress firmly. Bake for 30 minutes.

Remove the foil and continue baking about 35 more minutes until the potatoes are tender. The top should be brown.

Invert on a serving plate. Serve hot. Can be refrigerated overnight.

MAKES 6 TO 8 SERVINGS

Mashed Sweet Potatoes

ingredients

5 medium sweet potatoes

¼ cup butter or margarine

Salt to taste

Freshly grated nutmeg

Cook the sweet potatoes in a large pot in water to cover until tender. Drain and peel the potatoes. Mash with a potato masher for coarse potatoes, adding butter at the same time. Add salt, and grate fresh nutmeg over potatoes. For a smoother and creamier texture, use a food processor.

MAKES 8 SERVINGS

Sweet Duchess Potatoes

ingredients

3 medium russet potatoes

2 tablespoons butter

2 tablespoons low fat mayonnaise

Salt and freshly ground white
   pepper to taste

1 egg, beaten

1 20-ounce can sweet potatoes

¼ cup firmly packed brown sugar

¼ cup margarine

Preheat the oven to 400° and spray a 9x13-inch baking dish with nonstick spray. Wash and peel the russet potatoes. Slice and cook in salty water until tender. Mash thoroughly and add butter and the low fat mayonnaise. Season with white pepper. Beat until creamy, adding the egg.

Combine ¼ cup of syrup from the sweet potatoes with the sugar and margarine. Bring this to a boil, constantly stirring. Add the sweet potatoes and sauté until glazed.

Place the sweet potatoes in baking dish, leaving room between each piece. Spoon the russet potato mixture into a pastry tube and pipe a border around each sweet potato chunk. Bake for about 8 minutes.

SERVES 6 TO 8

Sweet Potato Purée

ingredients

4 medium sweet potatoes

3 tablespoons rum

Juice of 1 lime

3 tablespoons maple syrup

⅛ teaspoon ground cloves or 4 twists from nutmeg grinder

¼ teaspoon ground cinnamon

⅓ cup raisins

Butter

Cook the potatoes in a large pot in water to cover until tender. Drain, cool, and peel. (Or bake in the oven at 400° for 1 hour.) Mix the rum, lime juice, syrup, and spices in a small bowl. Stir in the raisins.

Preheat the oven to 350°. Butter an 8x11-inch baking dish. Mash the sweet potatoes with a potato masher or fork. Stir in the rum-raisin mixture. Place in the baking dish and cover with a few dots of butter. Bake for 15 minutes.

MAKES 6 SERVINGS

Madeira Casserole

ingredients

6 sweet potatoes

¼ cup butter, softened

½ cup half and half

½ cup Madeira wine

1 tablespoon orange rind, grated

½ teaspoon cinnamon

½ teaspoon freshly ground nutmeg

¼ teaspoon salt

Preheat the oven to 375° and spray a glass casserole dish with vegetable spray. Place the sweet potatoes on a baking sheet and bake for 1 hour.

Peel the sweet potatoes. Place in a food processor and purée. Add the softened butter, half and half, and Madeira, and mix well. Add the orange rind, cinnamon, nutmeg, and salt, and pulse the food processor. Pour the sweet potato mixture into the casserole dish. Reduce the heat to 300° and bake for 30 minutes.

Sherried Sweet Potatoes

ingredients

8 sweet potatoes

1 cup firmly packed brown sugar

2 tablespoons cornstarch

2 cups orange juice

½ teaspoon orange peel, grated

½ cup white raisins

6 tablespoons margarine or butter

⅓ cup sherry

¼ cup chopped pecans or walnuts

Cook the sweet potatoes in a large pot in water to cover until done. Cool and peel. Slice and arrange in a baking dish. Preheat the oven to 325°. Combine the brown sugar, cornstarch, orange juice, orange peel, raisins, margarine, and sherry in a saucepan, and cook until creamy, stirring constantly. Pour the sherry sauce over the sweet potatoes. Sprinkle with nuts. Bake for 30 minutes.

This dish can be made the day before and refrigerated.

MAKES 8 TO 10 SERVINGS

Bourbon Sweet Potatoes

ingredients

2 medium sweet potatoes

2 tablespoons bourbon

Wash and peel the sweet potatoes. Chop the sweet potatoes in a food processor until shredded. Spray a skillet with nonstick vegetable spray and sauté the sweet potatoes on low heat for 3 to 5 minutes until crisp-tender. Stir in the bourbon and allow to stand for at least 1 hour before serving.

MAKES 4 SERVINGS

Rum Sweet Potatoes

ingredients

3 sweet potatoes

2½ cups skim milk

3 eggs

2 cups sugar

½ cup slivered almonds

2 teaspoons ground cinnamon

½ cup rum

2 tablespoons margarine, cubed

Preheat the oven to 325°. Grate the raw sweet potatoes and place in a large bowl. Add milk immediately to prevent the sweet potatoes from turning dark. Beat the eggs in a small bowl and add to the mixture. Stir in the sugar gradually. Add the almonds and cinnamon, mixing well. Blend in the rum. Pour into a casserole dish and dot with margarine cubes. Bake for 2 hours.

MAKES 6 SERVINGS

For a slight variation, eliminate the cinnamon and instead of rum use one of the following liqueurs: creme de mint, creme de cacao, kahlua, brandy, or triple-sec.

Supreme Sweet Potatoes

ingredients

6 tablespoons butter or margarine

1 cup sugar

2 eggs, beaten well

½ cup milk

1½ teaspoons vanilla extract

½ teaspoon salt

3 cups sweet potato, cooked and
  mashed

Topping

1 cup brown sugar, packed

3 tablespoons margarine, melted

⅓ cup all-purpose flour

1 cup freshly grated coconut

Preheat the oven to 350°. Cream the butter and the sugar together in a large bowl. Add the beaten eggs, mixing well. Add the milk, vanilla, salt, and sweet potatoes. Pour into a greased baking dish.

Combine the brown sugar, melted margarine, flour, and coconut in a medium bowl. Mix together until crumbly using a pastry blender or fork. Sprinkle the topping over the sweet potatoes. Bake for 30 minutes.

May be prepared the day before and refrigerated before baking.

MAKES 8 SERVINGS

Sweet Potatoes Baked in Parchment

ingredients

3 medium sweet potatoes

3 11x16-inch sheets baking
   parchment

3 cloves garlic

3 sprigs rosemary or thyme

Salt and pepper to taste

3 tablespoons virgin olive oil

Preheat the oven to 400°. Wash and scrub the potatoes with a vegetable brush. Scar the outer skin of each sweet potato with a knife. Fold each piece of parchment paper in half. Place a sweet potato on each piece of paper. Top with a whole clove of garlic, a sprig of rosemary or thyme, salt, pepper, and 1 tablespoon of olive oil over each potato. Fold the paper over and roll tightly along the edges to form a pouch, giving a final twist at the ends to hold together. Bake the packages for 1 hour.

Open each package and remove the skin from each potato, being careful not to burn yourself with the steam. Serve immediately.

Grilled Sweet Potatoes

ingredients

4 medium sweet potatoes

4 tablespoons olive oil

4 cloves garlic, crushed

Salt and pepper to taste

Preheat the oven to 400°. Wash and scrub the sweet potatoes with a vegetable brush. Cut the sweet potatoes into diagonal slices about ⅓-inch thick. Toss with olive oil and crushed garlic. Sprinkle with salt and pepper. Place in a baking dish. Roast for 15 minutes.

Brush the slices lightly with olive oil and place on the grill. Use mesquite for lighter flavor or oak for a heavier flavor. If using charcoal, use sprigs of herbs over the charcoal for added flavor. Grill briefly until done.

Sweet Potatoes Au Gratin

ingredients

7 medium sweet potatoes

Salt and pepper to taste

1 tablespoon chopped thyme

1½ cups heavy cream

1 tablespoon cornstarch

1 cup shredded Gruyere cheese

2 tablespoons grated Parmesan
   cheese

Boil the sweet potatoes in a large pot in water to cover for 5 minutes. Drain, cool, peel, and dice into 1-inch pieces. Preheat the oven to 350°. Spray a baking dish with nonstick vegetable spray. Place the sweet potatoes in the dish and season with salt, pepper, and thyme. Mix the cream and cornstarch together and pour over the sweet potatoes. Bake for 30 minutes. Sprinkle with cheeses. Bake for 15 minutes. Brown under the broiler for about 3 minutes.

Orange Candied Sweet Potatoes

ingredients

4 large sweet potatoes

½ cup water

1¼ cups firmly packed brown sugar

Cinnamon

4 tablespoons butter or margarine

8 pieces orange peel

Boil the sweet potatoes in a large pot in water to cover until tender. Peel the skin off. Slice very thin. Preheat the oven to 350°. Spray a baking dish with nonstick vegetable spray. Place a layer of sweet potatoes in the dish. Pour the water into the dish. Sprinkle with brown sugar and cinnamon. Place dots of butter over this layer or spray with vegetable spray. Complete with another layer, adding the orange peel to the sugar, cinnamon, and butter on the top layer. Bake for 30 minutes or until brown and candied.

MAKES 6 SERVINGS

Sweet Potato Pone

ingredients

4 cups grated raw sweet potato

1 cup firmly packed brown sugar

2 cups dark corn syrup

1 cup water

1 teaspoon orange rind, grated

1 teaspoon lemon rind, grated

1 cup chopped citron

¼ cup seedless raisins

1 teaspoon cinnamon

1 teaspoon powdered or chopped
   ginger

Preheat the oven to 350° and grease a baking dish. Mix together the sweet potato, sugar, and syrup. Mix in the water. Add the citrus peels, citron, raisins, cinnamon, and ginger, mixing well. Place in the baking dish. Bake for 45 minutes until a crust forms on top.

This may be served as is or with cream.

MAKES 6 SERVINGS

Peaches and Potatoes

ingredients

1 16-ounce can sweet potatoes

1 16-ounce can peach slices
  or pieces

¼ cup port

½ cup orange juice

Freshly grated nutmeg

6 to 8 graham crackers, crumbled

Preheat the oven to 350°. Rinse the canned sweet potatoes. Slice and place in a greased baking dish. Drain the peaches, saving the juice. Mash the peaches or coarsely grind in a food processor. Mix together the peaches, port, orange juice, and peach juice in a medium bowl. Pour over the sweet potatoes and sprinkle with nutmeg and crumbled graham crackers. Bake for 30 minutes.

This can be mixed together and refrigerated overnight for the flavors to blend. A great dish to make ahead for entertaining.

Yummy Yams

ingredients

4 pounds sweet potatoes, cooked
  and mashed

½ cup melted butter

⅓ cup firmly packed brown sugar

⅓ cup orange juice

¼ cup bourbon

¾ teaspoon salt

½ teaspoon apple pie spice

½ to ¾ cup pecan halves

Preheat the oven to 350°. Combine all of the ingredients except the pecans in a large mixing bowl, mixing well. Pour into a greased 2½-quart casserole dish. Arrange the pecans around the edge of the dish. Bake for 45 minutes.

MAKES 8 TO 10 SERVINGS

Candied Sweet Potatoes

ingredients

4 medium or 3 large sweet potatoes

½ cup melted butter

1 cup sugar

¼ cup water

Peel the potatoes and cut into 2-inch slices. Combine the butter, sugar, and water in an electric skillet. Add the sweet potatoes. Cover and simmer at 250° for 1 hour or until done, turning frequently.

MAKES 6 TO 8 SERVINGS

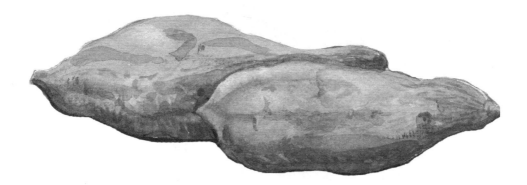

Highlands Apples and Sweet Potatoes

ingredients

5 medium sweet potatoes

2 tart apples

¾ teaspoon salt

½ cup firmly packed brown sugar

3 tablespoons butter

Preheat the oven to 375°. Wash the sweet potatoes, peel, and slice thinly. Wash the apples, peel, core, and slice. Arrange the apples and sweet potatoes in alternate layers in a buttered 1-quart casserole dish, sprinkling each layer of potatoes with salt and each layer of apples with brown sugar. Dot with butter and cover the casserole. Bake for about 45 minutes or until tender.

MAKES 6 SERVINGS

Banana Stuffed Sweet Potatoes

ingredients

8 small sweet potatoes

1 ripe banana

¼ cup orange juice

½ teaspoon freshly ground nutmeg

2 tablespoons firmly packed brown sugar

¼ teaspoon salt

¼ cup chopped unsalted peanuts

Preheat the oven to 300°. Scrub the sweet potatoes and pierce with a knife. Place on a baking sheet. Bake for 1 hour and 30 minutes. Let cool, then cut a thin lengthwise strip from end to end on each sweet potato. Scoop out the flesh. Purée the sweet potato with the banana in a food processor. Add the orange juice, nutmeg, brown sugar, and salt, and pulse the motor. Spoon the mixture into the potato skins. Arrange on a baking sheet. Sprinkle the chopped peanuts on top. Bake at 350° for 10 minutes or until hot.

MAKES 8 SERVINGS

Pineapple Stuffed Sweet Potatoes

ingredients

6 medium sweet potatoes

2 tablespoons butter

¼ teaspoon salt

1 tablespoon dry sherry

¾ cup crushed pineapple

1 cup dry bread crumbs

Preheat the oven to 375°. Scrub the sweet potatoes and spray lightly with nonstick vegetable spray. Place on a baking sheet and bake for 55 minutes or until tender.

Cut the sweet potatoes lengthwise into halves and scrape out the pulp. Purée the sweet potatoes with the butter, salt, and sherry in a food processor. Add the pineapple and pulse. Fill the shells and top with the dry bread crumbs. Spray thoroughly with nonstick butter spray. Place under a preheated broiler until crusty, about 3 minutes.

MAKES 6 SERVINGS

Walnut and Bourbon
Stuffed Sweet Potatoes

ingredients

6 small sweet potatoes

⅓ cup firmly packed brown sugar

2 tablespoons butter

3 tablespoons bourbon

½ teaspoon freshly ground nutmeg

¼ cup black walnuts

Preheat the oven to 300°. Scrub the sweet potatoes, spray with nonstick butter spray, and place on a baking sheet. Bake in the middle of the oven for 1 hour and 30 minutes. After 1 hour puncture the middle of each potato with a knife.

Cut the sweet potatoes lengthwise from end to end. Scrape the pulp out. Purée the pulp with the sugar, butter, bourbon, and nutmeg in a food processor. Fill the shells with the mixture and top with black walnuts. Spray with the butter spray and place under the broiler for 3 to 5 minutes until crusty.

MAKES 6 SERVINGS

Scarlett's Turnips and Sweet Potatoes

ingredients

6 small sweet potatoes

4 medium turnip roots

1 cup whole milk

1 cup heavy cream

⅓ cup minced onion

¼ teaspoon salt

Freshly ground white pepper

Freshly ground nutmeg

½ cup freshly grated Parmesan

¼ cup freshly grated Romano

Preheat the oven to 400° and spray a 2-quart au gratin dish with vegetable spray. Wash and peel the sweet potatoes and turnips. Cut crosswise into ¼-inch slices. Cook the sweet potatoes, turnips, milk, cream, and onion in a large pot on high heat until just before a rolling boil. Reduce the heat and simmer for 5 minutes.

Add the salt, pepper, and nutmeg. Remove from the heat. Spoon the sweet potato and turnip mixture into the au gratin dish and sprinkle the top with the grated cheeses. Bake for 40 to 45 minutes.

MAKES 6 TO 8 SERVINGS

Italian Grilled Sweet Potatoes

ingredients

2 medium sweet potatoes

1 red bell pepper

1 yellow bell pepper

1 green bell pepper

2 Vidalia onions

Fresh rosemary sprigs

Wash and peel the sweet potatoes. Cut into 2-inch cubes. Cover with water in a saucepan and cook for 12 minutes after coming to a boil. Drain. Wash, core, and slice in strips the peppers and Vidalia onions. Place on foil with fresh rosemary and spray with vegetable spray. Bake over coals until done. This dish may also be baked in the oven at 300°.

Sweet Potato Special

ingredients

5 pounds sweet potatoes

1 12-ounce package pitted prunes

1 cup water

2 cups fresh pineapple

¼ cup firmly packed dark
   brown sugar

1 tablespoon butter, diced

Cook the potatoes in a large pot in water to cover until they are soft. Drain the potatoes, pierce them with a fork, peel, and mash in a large bowl.

Preheat the oven to 350°. Cook the prunes in the water in a small saucepan for 5 minutes. Add the prunes, their cooking liquid, and the pineapple to the potatoes, mixing the ingredients to combine well. Place the potato mixture in a large ovenproof casserole. Sprinkle the potatoes with brown sugar and top with dots of butter. Place the uncovered casserole in the hot oven and bake for 20 minutes until the potatoes are heated through.

Can be prepared two days ahead for baking—bring to room temperature before baking.

Sweet Potato and Red Pepper Kugel

ingredients

4 large sweet potatoes, peeled

1 onion, quartered

1½ cups parsley sprigs

½ cup finely chopped almonds

1 large red bell pepper, cored
   and chopped

2 eggs

2 egg whites

¾ cup chicken broth

3 tablespoons vegetable oil

½ teaspoon salt

¾ teaspoon freshly ground white
   pepper

Preheat the oven to 350°. Spray a 2½-quart baking dish with nonstick vegetable spray. Cut the sweet potatoes into 2-inch chunks. Place in a food processor with the onion and chop coarsely. Add the parsley and process to chop the sweet potatoes finely. Combine the sweet potato mixture, almonds, red bell pepper, eggs, egg whites, chicken broth, oil, salt, and pepper in a large bowl. Mix thoroughly. Spoon into the prepared baking dish. Spray lightly with vegetable spray. Cover with foil and bake for 1 hour. Remove the foil and bake for an additional 15 minutes so that the kugel can brown.

MAKES 6 TO 8 SERVINGS

Roasted Sweet Potatoes with Garlic

ingredients

2 medium sweet potatoes, washed
and scrubbed

1½ tablespoons olive oil

2 large cloves garlic, sliced thin

Salt and pepper to taste

Slice the sweet potatoes in very thin rounds. Toss on a baking sheet with olive oil, garlic, salt, and pepper. Roast at 475° in the middle of the oven, stirring occasionally, about 30 minutes or until crisp.

This recipe can be used with any herb—rosemary or tarragon, for example.

Sweet Potato Soufflé

ingredients

¼ cup butter

¼ cup all-purpose flour

⅔ cup milk

2 cups puréed canned sweet
potatoes

4 eggs, beaten

Salt and freshly ground white
pepper to taste

Preheat the oven to 350°. Melt the butter in a heavy saucepan. Gradually add the flour. Slowly pour the milk in, stirring constantly to remove all lumps. Cook until well blended. Add the sweet potatoes and blend. Add 1 cup of the cooked sweet potato mixture to the beaten eggs, making sure not to scramble the eggs. Add this to the remaining sweet potato mixture. Season with salt and pepper. Beat the egg whites until stiff and fold into the mixture. Pour into a buttered soufflé dish and bake for 35 minutes or until set.

Sweet Potato Surprise

ingredients

2 cups puréed canned sweet
  potatoes

1 egg, beaten

¼ teaspoon salt

Pepper to taste

12 miniature marshmallows

½ cup crushed corn flakes

2 tablespoons butter, unsalted

Combine the sweet potato purée and beaten egg in a large bowl. Season with salt and pepper. Shape some of the mixture around each marshmallow to form a small ball. Roll in crushed corn flakes. Melt the butter in a skillet and sauté the balls until crisp. Serve immediately.

MAKES 12 BALLS

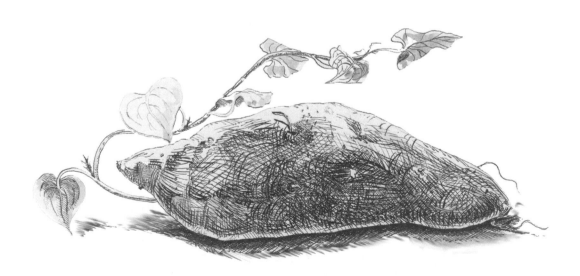

Crusty Sweet Potatoes

ingredients

1 medium can sweet potato slices

6 tablespoons unsalted butter

¼ cup sugar

Salt to taste

Drain the sweet potato slices and place on paper towels to dry. Melt the butter in a large skillet and place the sweet potato slices flat down in the bottom. Sprinkle with sugar. Cook over low heat about 15 minutes, turning them once. Season with salt.

Curried Fruit and Sweet Potatoes

ingredients

1 16-ounce can sweet potatoes
1 16-ounce can pear halves
1 16-ounce can peach halves
1 16-ounce can pineapple chunks
1 6-ounce jar maraschino cherries
2 teaspoons curry powder

Open and drain the sweet potatoes and pears. Pour off half the peach, pineapple, and cherry juices. Pour the remaining juices, fruit, and sweet potatoes in a large pot. Add the curry powder. Bring to just below boiling point over high heat. Immediately reduce the heat and simmer for 15 minutes.

This can be mixed the day before serving to allow the curry powder to marry better.

Great to serve with a quiche. This is one of my favorite side dishes to serve for a hot winter brunch.

Sweet Potato
desserts

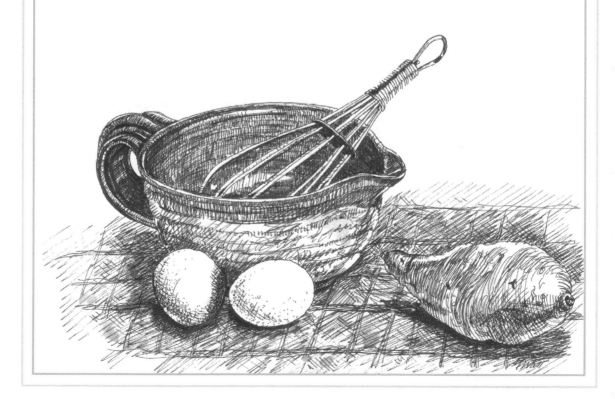

Southern Holiday Pudding

ingredients

3 medium sweet potatoes

2 cups milk

¾ cup Tennessee whiskey
  or bourbon

3 eggs

2 cups sugar

2 tablespoons butter or margarine,
  softened

¾ cup blanched, slivered almonds

Preheat the oven to 325° and spray a casserole dish with nonstick vegetable spray. Boil the sweet potatoes in a large pot in water to cover until tender. Drain and cool. Peel by pulling the skin away. Place in a food processor and purée. Add the milk and whiskey, mixing well. Beat the eggs in a medium bowl, adding sugar gradually. Add to the sweet potato mixture. Mix in the butter. Stir in the almonds. Spread the sweet potato mixture in the prepared pan. Bake for 1 hour.

Sweet Potato Pound Cake

ingredients

1 cup unsalted butter or margarine, softened

2 cups sugar

1 16-ounce can sweet potatoes, drained

1 teaspoon vanilla extract

4 eggs

3 cups cake flour

2 teaspoons baking powder

½ teaspoon baking soda

1 teaspoon ground cinnamon

½ teaspoon freshly ground nutmeg

¼ teaspoon salt

Glaze

1 cup sifted confectioners' sugar

1 tablespoon orange juice

1 tablespoon shredded orange peel

Preheat the oven to 350°. Cream together the butter and sugar in a food processor until light and fluffy. Add the sweet potatoes and vanilla and mix until the sweet potatoes are completely puréed. Add the eggs, one at a time, pulsing after each addition. Combine the flour, baking powder, baking soda, cinnamon, nutmeg, and salt in a large mixing bowl and sift together. Slowly add the flour mixture to the sweet potato mixture, blending well.

Spray a 10-inch tube pan with nonstick vegetable spray. Pour the batter into the tube pan. Bake for 1 hour and 20 minutes or until a wooden toothpick inserted in the center comes out clean. Cool the cake in the pan on a wire rack, then invert onto a serving plate.

To make the Glaze

Stir together the sifted confectioners' sugar, orange juice, and orange peel in a small bowl. Spoon the glaze over the cake so that it drizzles down the side.

Sweet Potato Cookies

ingredients

2 cups canned sweet potatoes, drained

2 cups all-purpose flour

½ teaspoon salt

1 cup plus 4 tablespoons margarine or unsalted butter

¾ cup finely chopped walnuts or pecans

¼ cup firmly packed brown sugar

Preheat the oven to 350°. Spray a cookie sheet with nonstick vegetable spray. Purée the sweet potatoes in a food processor. Mix together the sweet potatoes, flour, salt, and 1 cup of margarine in a large bowl to form a dough. Roll the dough into a thin sheet on a lightly floured pastry cloth. Cut with a floured cookie cutter in circle shapes.

Mix together the nuts, remaining margarine, and brown sugar in a small bowl. Place a teaspoonful of this nut mixture on one half of each cookie circle. Fold over the other half of the dough and crimp the edges together to seal them. Place the cookies on the cookie sheet. Bake for about 12 to 20 minutes until brown.

MAKES 24 COOKIES

Sweet Potato Doughnuts

ingredients

1½ cups cooked, puréed sweet
  potatoes

2 eggs

¼ cup butter, melted

2 tablespoons orange extract
  flavoring

⅓ cup plain yogurt

½ cup walnuts or pecans

3 cups self-rising flour

¼ teaspoon freshly grated nutmeg

2½ teaspoons cinnamon, divided

¾ cup brown sugar

1 teaspoon grated orange rind

1 teaspoon grated orange rind

Vegetable oil for frying

½ cup granulated sugar

Combine the sweet potato, eggs, butter, orange flavoring, and yogurt; beat until smooth. Using the metal blade of a food processor, grind the nuts into very small pieces.

Sift the flour, nutmeg, and 1 teaspoon cinnamon into a large mixing bowl; add the brown sugar, nuts, and grated orange rind; mix well. Stir the sweet potato mixture into the flour mixture, mixing to a soft dough. Knead dough on a lightly floured surface until smooth, adding more flour if mixture becomes too sticky. Roll the dough out and cut into doughnut rounds with a cutter. Place doughnuts on raised cookie sheets and refrigerate until firm.

Deep fry the doughnuts in hot vegetable oil until browned; remove from oil and place on paper towels. When lightly cooled, roll doughnuts in combined sugar and remaining cinnamon.

MAKES ABOUT 35 DOUGHNUTS

Tea Party Madeleines

ingredients

¾ cup cooked sweet potatoes

2 eggs, well beaten

1 cup sugar

1 tablespoon freshly squeezed
   lemon juice

¾ cup butter, melted

1 cup cake flour, sifted

2 tablespoons confectioners' sugar

Preheat the oven to 350°. Spray 24 large or 50 miniature madeleine molds with nonstick spray. Purée the sweet potatoes in a food processor.

Heat the eggs and sugar in the top of a double boiler over simmering water until just lukewarm. Immediately beat until fluffy. After the mixture has cooled add the lemon juice and puréed sweet potatoes, blending well. Blend in the butter. Add the sifted cake flour and mix well. Spoon the batter into the molds. Bake for about 10 to 12 minutes until golden brown.

Cool on a cake rack. Remove the madeleines from the molds and sprinkle with confectioners' sugar.

MAKES 24 LARGE OR 50 MINIATURE MADELEINES

This French tea cake was made famous by Marcel Proust.

Sweet Potato Custard
with Orange Cream

ingredients

1½ cups cooked puréed sweet
   potato

⅓ cup granulated sugar

1 egg

2 egg yolks

⅛ teaspoon cinnamon

⅛ teaspoon nutmeg

⅛ teaspoon allspice

⅛ teaspoon confectioner's sugar

½ teaspoon grated orange rind

⅔ cup heavy cream

3 medium oranges in individual
   sections

Orange Cream Sauce

½ cup sour cream

2 teaspoons Grand Marnier

2 teaspoons confectioners' sugar

Purée cooked sweet potatoes a smooth consistency with no lumps left. Mix sugar, egg, egg yolks, spices, and orange rind together. Blend in sweet potatoes and cream. Divide mixture between 6 ovenproof dishes.

Place dishes in baking pan with enough boiling water to come halfway up the sides of the serving dishes. Bake uncovered at 325° for 45 minutes to one hour. Custard is done when knife inserted in the middle of the custard comes out clean. Cool, then refrigerate until cold. Serve with orange cream sauce, orange segments, and sprinkled confectioners' sugar.

Pineapple Sweet Potato
Praline Pudding

ingredients

1 16-ounce can sweet potatoes,
drained

4 tablespoons margarine or
unsalted butter

4 egg yolks

3 tablespoons firmly packed brown
sugar

2 tablespoons freshly grated
orange rind

3 tablespoons rum

1 14-ounce can crushed unsweetened pineapple

¼ teaspoon freshly ground nutmeg

½ teaspoon ground ginger

Salt and white pepper to taste

Nonstick vegetable spray

Topping

½ cup margarine or
unsalted butter

1 cup firmly packed
brown sugar

1 cup shredded coconut

1 cup pecan pieces

2 tablespoons rum

¼ cup light cream

Preheat the oven to 350°. Drain the potatoes and purée in a food processor. Add the margarine or butter, egg yolks, and brown sugar, and blend until smooth. Add the orange rind, rum, and pineapple, and mix well. Add the nutmeg, ginger, salt, and pepper. Spray a 2-quart baking dish with the vegetable spray. Pour the sweet potato mixture into the baking dish.

To make the Topping

In a medium bowl cream the butter and brown sugar together until smooth. Fold in the coconut, pecans, rum and cream.

Spread the mixture evenly over the sweet potato mixture. Bake for 30 minutes. Run under the broiler until the topping begins to bubble.

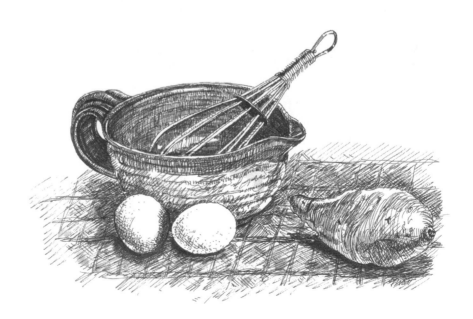

Pumpkin and Sweet Potato Pie

ingredients

1 unbaked 9-inch pie shell

1 cup canned sweet potatoes

1 cup canned pumpkin

¼ cup margarine or butter, softened

¾ cup sugar

½ teaspoon freshly ground nutmeg

¼ teaspoon ground ginger

¼ teaspoon ground cloves

¼ teaspoon ground cinnamon

¼ teaspoon ground allspice

¼ teaspoon salt

3 eggs

1 12-ounce can evaporated milk

Prebake each empty pie shell as directed on the package. Preheat the oven to 350°. In the bowl of an electric mixer combine and blend together the sweet potatoes, pumpkin, butter, sugar, and spices. Add the eggs one at a time, mixing well after each addition. Add the evaporated milk to the mixture and pour into the prebaked pie shell. Bake for about 1 hour until done.

MAKES 6 TO 8 SERVINGS

Easy Sweet Potato Pie

ingredients

1½ cups canned sweet potatoes,
   drained
¾ cup sugar
½ cup firmly packed brown sugar
½ cup margarine
1 tablespoon vanilla extract
2 eggs
1 14-ounce can sweetened
   condensed milk
2 tablespoons all-purpose flour
1 teaspoon baking powder
½ teaspoon freshly grated nutmeg
½ teaspoon cinnamon
2 9-inch unbaked pie shells

Preheat the oven to 425°. In a food processor purée the sweet potatoes. Add the sugar, brown sugar, and margarine, and process until creamy. Add the vanilla, eggs, and condensed milk, and beat until smooth. In a separate bowl combine the flour, baking powder, nutmeg, and cinnamon. Add the dry ingredients to the sweet potato mixture and mix well. Divide among the pie crusts. Place on a baking sheet. Bake for 40 to 45 minutes.

MAKES 12 SERVINGS

Sweet Potato Lime Cake

ingredients

½ cup soft butter

1 teaspoon grated lime peel or zest

⅔ cup granulated sugar

2 eggs

¾ cup cooked sweet potato, puréed

1½ cups self-rising flour

¼ cup all-purpose flour

¼ cup milk

⅔ tablespoon confectioners' sugar

Preheat the oven to 350°.

Spray a tube pan with nonstick baking spray with flour. Cream butter, lime peel, and sugar with an electric mixer until light and fluffy. Add eggs one at a time bearing after each one. Stir in sweet potatoes. Sift flours together and add sweet potato mixture and milk alternately, blending well. Pour mixture into prepared pan and spread evenly. Bake for about 40 minutes until done when a toothpick comes out clean. Cool on wire rack and then remove from pan. Sprinkle with confectioners' sugar.

Tropical Sweet Potato Cake

ingredients

3 medium sweet potatoes, peeled
   and thickly sliced

2 tablespoons butter

¾ cup brown sugar

¼ cup dark rum

4 eggs

½ cup milk

2 teaspoons grated lime rind

1 tablespoon lime juice

½ teaspoon ground cinnamon

½ teaspoon ground nutmeg

½ teaspoon salt

2 teaspoons baking powder

Preheat oven to 350° and spray a 9x5-inch loaf pan with nonstick vegetable spray.

Cook sweet potatoes in enough water to cover until tender, 20 to 25 minutes. Drain and purée in a food processor.

Mix in butter, sugar, and rum while the potatoes are still warm.

Beat in the eggs, one at a time.

Add the milk, grated rind, and lime juice.

Sift together the cinnamon, nutmeg, salt, and baking powder. Add to the sweet potato mixture and mix thoroughly.

Pour into the loaf pan.

Bake for about 1 hour or until a toothpick comes out clean.

Let cool five minutes, then turn onto a rack to finish cooling.

SERVES 4

Sweet Potato Cobbler

ingredients

Filling

8 large sweet potatoes, peeled and
   sliced

2 cups granulated sugar plus
   1 teaspoon for sprinkling

1 teaspoon cinnamon

¼ teaspoon allspice

¼ teaspoon nutmeg

½ cup butter

1 teaspoon vanilla extract

Crust

3 cups all-purpose flour

1 teaspoon salt

¾ cup shortening

6 to 8 tablespoons ice water

Preheat the oven to 350°. Combine the flour and salt. Blend in the shortening using a pastry blender. Slowly stir in ice water, spoon by spoon, to hold the dough together. Divide the dough into two equal pieces and press out to 4 to 5 inches. Wrap tightly and refrigerate.

Mix the sliced sweet potatoes, 2 cups sugar, spices, and butter in a saucepan. Add enough water to just cover and bring to a boil. Reduce the temperature and cook about 12 to 15 minutes until sweet potatoes are tender. Set aside to cool. When cool, stir in vanilla extract.

Spray an 8x12-inch glass baking dish with nonstick vegetable spray. Roll out one crust to ⅛-inch thick. Cut dough into 2-inch strips and line the baking dish. Pour filling into dish, covering crust pieces. Roll out second piece of dough into 9x13-inch crust and place on top of baking dish. Trim edges, cut 3 to 4 slits to vent the cobbler, and sprinkle with the remaining sugar. Bake until golden brown, about 40 to 50 minutes.

Date Nut Sweet Potato Squares

ingredients

1½ cups canned sweet potatoes, drained

1 cup margarine, softened

2 cups firmly packed brown sugar

2 eggs

1 teaspoon vanilla extract

¼ cup milk or water

2½ cups all-purpose flour

1½ teaspoons baking powder

½ teaspoon salt

½ teaspoon ground cloves

½ teaspoon freshly grated nutmeg

½ teaspoon cinnamon

1 pound pitted dried dates

1¼ cups slivered almonds

Preheat the oven to 350° and spray a 9x13-inch baking pan with nonstick vegetable spray. Purée the sweet potatoes in a food processor. Cream the margarine and sugar in a large bowl with an electric mixer, and add the eggs and vanilla. Add this and the water or milk to the puréed sweet potatoes and beat well. Sift together the flour, baking powder, salt, cloves, nutmeg, and cinnamon in a separate bowl. Cut the pitted dates and almonds into thirds and toss with ¼ cup of the flour mixture. Gradually add the remaining flour mixture to the sweet potato mixture and blend. Fold in the dates and almonds. Pour the batter into the baking pan. Bake for 60 minutes or until a wooden toothpick inserted in the center comes out clean.

Cool on a cake rack, cut into squares, and remove from pan.

MAKES 12 SERVINGS

Lime Sweet Potato Chiffon Pie

ingredients

2 cups canned sweet potatoes,
   drained

¼ cup firmly packed brown sugar

¼ cup margarine, melted

4 eggs, separated

½ teaspoon salt

¼ teaspoon nutmeg

⅛ teaspoon cloves

1 cup heavy (whipping) cream

3 tablespoons freshly squeezed
   lime juice

1 teaspoon freshly grated lime rind

1 tablespoon sugar

1 9-inch pie crust, partially baked

Preheat the oven to 400°. Purée the sweet potatoes in a food processor. Cream together the brown sugar and margarine in a large bowl. Add the egg yolks, salt, spices, cream, lime juice, and rind, and beat well. Beat in the puréed sweet potatoes until smooth. Beat the egg whites in a separate bowl with sugar until they form stiff peaks. Stir half the beaten egg whites into the sweet potato mixture until completely mixed together. Fold in the remaining egg whites. Pour into a partially baked pie crust. Bake for 10 minutes.

Reduce the heat to 325° and continue baking for about 45 minutes until done. Cool and chill. Serve cold.

MAKES 6 TO 8 SERVINGS

Sweet Potato Brownies

ingredients

1 cup canned sweet potatoes

1 egg

1 egg white

½ cup margarine, melted

1 cup firmly packed brown sugar

1 tablespoon vanilla extract

2 cups all-purpose flour

½ teaspoon baking powder

½ teaspoon salt

¼ teaspoon ground cloves

¼ teaspoon allspice

¼ teaspoon mace

¼ cup milk, as needed

Frosting

1½ ounces cream cheese, softened

3 tablespoons margarine, softened

1 tablespoon vanilla extract

1 cup confectioners' sugar, sifted

Milk, a few drops if needed

1 cup chopped nuts (optional)

Preheat the oven to 350°. Spray a 9x13-inch baking pan with nonstick vegetable spray. Purée the sweet potatoes in a food processor. Cream together the egg and egg white, margarine, brown sugar, and vanilla in a large bowl. Add the puréed sweet potato and beat until smooth and creamy. In a separate bowl sift together the flour, baking powder, salt, cloves, allspice, and mace. Slowly add the dry ingredients to the sweet potato mixture alternately with the milk, stirring just until combined. Pour the batter into the baking pan and cook for 25 minutes or until a wooden toothpick inserted into the center comes out clean. Cool completely on a wire rack.

To make the Frosting

Combine the cream cheese, margarine, vanilla, and confectioners' sugar in a medium bowl, and beat until smooth and creamy. Add drops of milk only if needed to reach the right consistency for spreading. If using nuts, add just before spreading on the cooled brownies. Cut into 2-inch squares and store in the refrigerator.

Gingerbread Yummies

ingredients

½ cup skim milk

½ teaspoon lemon juice

2 tablespoons applesauce

½ cup packed brown sugar

¼ cup cholesterol-free egg
   substitute

2 cups all-purpose flour

1½ teaspoons baking soda

1½ teaspoons ground ginger

1 teaspoon ground cinnamon

1 cup water

½ cup molasses

¼ cup puréed cooked sweet
   potatoes

Preheat the oven to 350°. Combine the milk and lemon juice in a large bowl. Add the applesauce, brown sugar, and egg substitute, and mix well. Set aside. Combine the flour, baking soda, ginger, and cinnamon in a separate bowl. Set aside. Combine the water, molasses, and sweet potatoes in a separate bowl. Add the flour mixture alternately with the sweet potato mixture to the applesauce mixture, beginning and ending with flour mixture. The batter will be lumpy. Do not overmix.

Spray a 9-inch square pan with nonstick cooking spray. Pour the batter into the prepared pan. Bake for 40 to 45 minutes or until a toothpick inserted in the center comes out clean. Cool in the pan on a wire rack.

Serve with nondairy whipped topping if desired.

MAKES 8 SERVINGS

—*Sweet Potato Council of the U.S., Inc.*

Heavenly Cheesecake Bars

ingredients

1 cup all-purpose flour

⅓ cup firmly packed brown sugar

5 tablespoons butter

½ cup finely chopped walnuts or pecans

1 8-ounce package cream cheese, softened

¾ cup sugar

½ cup mashed cooked sweet potatoes

2 eggs

1½ teaspoons cinnamon

1 teaspoon allspice

1 teaspoon vanilla extract

Preheat the oven to 350°. Combine the flour and brown sugar in a medium bowl. Using a pastry blender or two knives, cut in the butter to make a crumb mixture. Stir in the nuts. Set aside ¾ cup of the mixture for topping. Press the remaining mixture into the bottom of an 8-inch square baking pan. Bake for 15 minutes. Cool slightly.

Combine the cream cheese, sugar, sweet potatoes, eggs, cinnamon, allspice, and vanilla in a large mixing bowl. Blend until smooth. Pour over the baked crust. Sprinkle with the reserved topping. Bake for an additional 30 to 35 minutes. Cool then cut into bars.

MAKES 32 1x2-INCH BARS

—*Sweet Potato Council of the U.S., Inc.*

Bourbon Sweet Potato Cake

ingredients

2 cups canned sweet potatoes,
  drained

3 cups cake flour

3 teaspoons baking powder

1 teaspoon salt

½ teaspoon nutmeg

1 teaspoon cinnamon

1 cup unsalted butter

½ cup sugar

1¼ cups firmly packed brown sugar

5 eggs, separated

⅓ cup milk

2 tablespoons bourbon

1 cup chopped nuts

¼ teaspoon cream of tartar

Preheat the oven to 350°. Line the bottom of a tube pan with waxed paper and spray with nonstick vegetable spray. Purée the drained sweet potatoes in a food processor. Sift together the flour, baking powder, salt, and spices in a medium bowl. Cream the butter and sugars together in a separate bowl. Add the egg yolks to the butter and sugar mixture, one at a time, and beat. Add the milk gradually, and beat for 2 to 3 minutes. Add the sifted dry ingredients to this gradually, stirring well. Add the bourbon and nuts. Blend in the puréed sweet potatoes in a separate bowl. In a separate bowl, beat the egg whites until they form stiff peaks, adding the cream of tartar when the egg whites are foamy. Fold the egg whites into the sweet potato mixture. Pour the batter into the tube pan. Bake for 1 hour or until done. Cool on a cake rack.

MAKES 8 TO 10 SERVINGS

Sweet Potato Cake

ingredients

1 cup all-purpose flour

1 teaspoon baking soda

½ teaspoon salt

½ teaspoon nutmeg

½ teaspoon cinnamon

¼ cup butter

⅔ cup sugar

1 egg

1 teaspoon vanilla extract

1 large apple, peeled and grated

1 sweet potato, peeled and grated

½ cup chopped nuts

Preheat the oven to 350° and grease an 8- or 9-inch square baking pan. Sift together the flour, baking soda, salt, nutmeg, and cinnamon in a medium bowl. Cream together the butter and sugar in a large bowl. Beat in the egg and vanilla. Stir in the apple and sweet potato. Add the flour mixture and stir together well. Stir in the nuts. Pour into the greased baking pan. Bake for 35 to 40 minutes.

Let the cake cool on a rack for 10 minutes. Turn the cake over and finish cooling.

MAKES 8 SERVINGS

Christmas Pudding

ingredients

½ cup margarine, melted

½ cup sugar

3 eggs, separated and beaten

2 cups milk

1 cup water

2 cups grated raw sweet potato

⅛ teaspoon ground cinnamon
   or to taste

⅛ teaspoon ground cloves or to taste

¼ teaspoon ground nutmeg
   or to taste

½ cup citron

½ cup raisins

½ cup currants

All-purpose flour

Hard Sauce

½ cup butter

1 cup sugar

¼ cup brandy, bourbon, or whiskey

1 egg white

Freshly grated nutmeg

Preheat the oven to 350° and grease a baking dish. Cream the margarine and sugar together in a large bowl. Add the egg yolks to the sugar mixture, mixing well. Gradually add the milk and water, beating thoroughly. Add the grated sweet potato and mix well. Add the cinnamon, cloves, and nutmeg. Dredge the fruit in flour and add to the sweet potato mixture. Fold in the stiffly beaten egg whites. Pour into the baking dish. Bake for 1 hour and 30 minutes. Serve with Hard Sauce.

To make the Hard Sauce

Cream the butter and sugar in a medium bowl. Add the brandy and mix well. Blend in the egg white. Serve over the Christmas Pudding and sprinkle with nutmeg.

MAKES 6 SERVINGS

Holiday Casserole

ingredients

2 cups cooked, mashed sweet
  potatoes
1 cup sugar
1 egg
½ cup grated coconut
1 teaspoon vanilla extract
1 cup evaporated milk
Salt to taste

Glaze

1 cup sugar
2 tablespoons cornstarch
1 15-ounce can crushed pineapple
  and juice
1 8-ounce bottle Maraschino
  cherries and juice

Preheat the oven to 350°. In a large bowl combine the sweet potatoes, 1 cup of sugar, egg, coconut, vanilla, and evaporated milk in a large bowl. Season with salt. Pour into a greased baking dish. Bake for 45 minutes.

To make the Glaze

Combine 1 cup of sugar, the cornstarch, pineapple and juice, and cherries and juice in a saucepan. Cook until the consistency of syrup. Pour over the potato mixture and bake for 10 more minutes.

MAKES 6 SERVINGS

Sweet Potato Cobbler

ingredients

Pastry for double-crust 9-inch pie

3 cups sliced, cooked sweet
  potatoes

1 cup sugar

Butter

1 teaspoon ground nutmeg

½ teaspoon ground cinnamon

1¼ cups water

Preheat the oven to 350°. On a lightly floured surface roll out two-thirds of the crust. Place in the bottom of an ungreased 10-inch square baking dish or 9-inch skillet. Combine the sweet potatoes and sugar in a large bowl. Arrange in the bottom of the pie crust. Roll out the remaining pastry and cut into strips. Layer the strips across the pan in a lattice pattern. Dot with butter and sprinkle with nutmeg and cinnamon. Pour the water over the top of the dish. Bake for 45 to 60 minutes.

MAKES 8 SERVINGS

Sweet Potato Spice Cake

ingredients

1 cup canned sweet potatoes

1 18¼-ounce box yellow cake mix

½ cup vegetable oil

¾ cup firmly packed brown sugar

½ teaspoon freshly ground nutmeg

1 teaspoon ground cinnamon

½ teaspoon ground allspice

4 eggs

Glaze

¼ cup margarine or unsalted butter

½ cup firmly packed brown sugar

½ cup walnuts

Preheat the oven to 350°. Spray a 10-inch bundt pan with nonstick vegetable spray. Purée the canned sweet potatoes in a food processor. Combine the cake mix, sweet potatoes, oil, ¾ cup of brown sugar, and spices in a large mixing bowl. Beat for 1 minute with an electric mixer on high. Add the eggs, one at a time, mixing after each addition. Beat 2 minutes more on medium speed. Pour into the bundt pan.

To make the Glaze

Cream the butter with ½ cup of brown sugar in a medium bowl. Add the nuts.

Pour half of the mixture on top of the cake batter. Bake for 1 hour or until a wooden toothpick inserted in the center comes out clean. Cool the cake in the pan on a cake rack for about 20 minutes.

Invert the pan on top of a serving plate. Remove and drizzle the remaining glaze on the cake.

Sweet Potato Roll

ingredients

3 eggs

1 cup sugar

1 teaspoon lemon juice

⅔ cup canned puréed sweet potato

¾ cup cake flour

1 teaspoon baking powder

½ teaspoon ground cinnamon

1 teaspoon ground ginger

½ teaspoon freshly ground nutmeg

¼ teaspoon salt

Preheat the oven to 375°. Line a jelly roll pan with waxed paper. Spray the waxed paper with nonstick vegetable spray. Beat the eggs in a large bowl with an electric mixer on high for about 3 minutes or until frothy. Add the sugar, lemon juice, and sweet potato. Mix until blended. Combine the flour, baking powder, cinnamon, ginger, nutmeg, and salt in a large bowl. Add the dry ingredients to the sweet potato mixture and beat on low speed until smooth. Pour the batter into the jelly roll pan and spread evenly. Bake for about 15 minutes until done.

Filling

1 8-ounce package cream cheese, softened

4 tablespoons butter, softened

¾ cup confectioners' sugar

1 teaspoon vanilla extract

1 cup drained crushed pineapple

To make the Filling

Combine the cream cheese, butter, confectioners' sugar, and vanilla in a medium bowl, beating until smooth. Add the crushed pineapple and mix by hand until blended.

Immediately remove the cake from the pan by inverting onto a tea towel sprinkled with confectioners' sugar. Roll into a roll, leaving the waxed paper on the cake. Unroll, remove the waxed paper, and spread with filling. Immediately reroll the cake. Let cool completely and refrigerate for about 1 hour before serving. Slice when ready to serve.

Sweet Potato Logs

ingredients

4 medium sweet potatoes, cooked
and mashed

1 teaspoon vanilla extract

1 cup sugar

1 egg, beaten

¼ cup milk

3 tablespoons all-purpose flour plus
extra for dredging raisins

1 teaspoon ground cinnamon

½ cup chopped pecans

½ cup raisins

1 cup grated coconut

½ cup melted butter

Preheat the oven to 375° and grease a baking sheet. Combine the sweet potatoes, vanilla, sugar, egg, milk, flour, cinnamon, and pecans in a large bowl, mixing well. Dredge the raisins in the extra flour. Add the raisins to the sweet potato mixture, mixing well. Cool the mixture. Shape into 8 logs or croquettes, and roll in coconut. Place on the baking sheet and drizzle the melted butter over the logs. Bake for about 20 minutes or until browned and crisp.

MAKES 8 SERVINGS

Sweet Potato Ice Cream

ingredients

3 eggs

1½ cups sugar

2 cups whole milk

1 teaspoon salt

1 teaspoon all-purpose flour

1 teaspoon vanilla extract

¼ teaspoon lemon extract

1 cup heavy cream

1 5-ounce can evaporated milk

1 cup cooked, mashed sweet
  potatoes

Whip the eggs and sugar together in a saucepan. Add the whole milk and salt, and simmer over low heat until heated. Whisk in the flour until well blended and thickened. Increase the heat and cook, stirring constantly, until the mixture is at the boiling point. Remove from the heat and add the vanilla and lemon extracts, heavy cream, evaporated milk, and mashed sweet potatoes. Strain to remove any lumps. Freeze in an ice cream freezer according to the manufacturers' directions.

MAKES ONE-HALF GALLON

This recipe is from Mr. Harold Hoecker, executive secretary of the Sweet Potato Council of the U.S., Inc.

Sweet Potato Candy

ingredients

2 cups cooked, mashed sweet
potatoes

1 cup crushed pineapple, undrained

½ teaspoon salt

¼ teaspoon cream of tartar

2 cups firmly packed brown sugar

⅔ cup boiling water

1 cup almonds, shelled

Combine the sweet potatoes, pineapple, and salt in a saucepan. Simmer for about 5 minutes, stirring constantly. Dissolve the cream of tartar and brown sugar in the boiling water. Add to the sweet potato mixture. Cook over low heat until a soft ball is formed when a drop is placed in cold water. Remove from the heat and beat until smooth and shiny. Mix in the almonds. Drop by a teaspoon onto a buttered surface.

MAKES 6 DOZEN PIECES

This recipe is from Mr. Harold Hoecker, executive secretary of the Sweet Potato Council of the U.S., Inc.

Sweet Potato Pralines

ingredients

1 cup buttermilk

1 cup margarine or butter

2½ cups sugar

2½ cups chopped pecans

2 tablespoons cooked, puréed sweet
potatoes

1 tablespoon vanilla extract

½ teaspoon baking soda

Mix the buttermilk, butter, and sugar in a saucepan. Cook over low heat, stirring constantly, until the sugar is dissolved. Add the pecans and cook over medium heat, stirring constantly, until a candy thermometer reads 239°. Add the puréed sweet potatoes, vanilla, and baking soda. Stir rapidly until the mixture is thick and creamy. Drop immediately by tablespoon onto waxed paper that has been sprayed with nonstick vegetable spray. Allow to cool and set.

This is an excellent recipe to use that small amount of leftover sweet potatoes.

Peanut Butter Candy Rolls

ingredients

1 medium sweet potato

1 tablespoon margarine or butter

1 teaspoon salt

1 teaspoon vanilla extract

3 16-ounce boxes confectioners' sugar

1 cup creamy peanut butter

Scrub the sweet potato and boil until tender. Cool and peel. Purée the sweet potato with the margarine in a food processor. Add the salt and vanilla, blending well. Set aside 2 tablespoons of confectioners' sugar to sprinkle on the pastry board. Add the remaining confectioners' sugar gradually until the mixture is the consistency of thick, cooked dough. Wrap in a tea towel and chill.

Use enough sweet potato mixture to roll out a circle ¼-inch thick and 12 inches in diameter. Keep the remaining sweet potato mixture covered with a damp tea towel. Heat the peanut butter in a saucepan, and spread in a thin layer over the rolled out sweet potato mixture. Roll like a jelly roll. Slice into 1-inch pieces, keeping the round shape. Prepare the remaining sweet potato mixture and peanut butter. Store the candy in a tightly covered container.

Bon Bon Sweet Potato Candy

ingredients

1 pound dried apricots or peaches,
  chopped

4 cups flaked coconut

2 cups chopped toasted pecans

1½ cups cooked, puréed sweet
  potatoes

2 16-ounce boxes confectioners'
  sugar

1 14-ounce can sweetened
  condensed milk

Combine all the ingredients in a large bowl. Chill covered for 2 hours. Shape into 1-inch balls. Store in a tightly covered container in the refrigerator.

Mississippi Sweet Potato Cake

ingredients

All-purpose flour

1 cup cooked, puréed sweet
  potatoes

4 eggs

1 18¼-ounce box spice cake mix

1 cup water

1 3-ounce box instant vanilla
  pudding mix

½ cup vegetable oil

Cream Cheese Filling

1 8-ounce package cream cheese,
  softened

2 tablespoons milk

2 tablespoons vanilla extract

Pinch salt

5 cups confectioners' sugar

1 cup chopped pecans

Preheat the oven to 350°. Spray three 8-inch round cake pans with nonstick vegetable spray. Sprinkle with flour. Mix the sweet potatoes, eggs, cake mix, water, pudding mix, and oil in a large bowl, and beat well. Pour into the prepared cake pans. Bake for 25 to 30 minutes.

To make the Filling

Blend the softened cream cheese, milk, vanilla, and salt in a large bowl. Gradually add the confectioners' sugar, beating until the frosting is smooth. Stir in the pecans. Spread between layers and on the top and sides of the cake.

Easy Caramel Sweet Potato Pie

ingredients

¼ cup margarine

1 7-ounce can coconut

½ cup chopped pecans

1½ cups cooked, puréed sweet potatoes

1 8-ounce package cream cheese, softened

1 14-ounce can sweetened condensed milk

2 8-ounce packages whipped topping, thawed

3 graham cracker crusts

1 12-ounce jar caramel ice cream topping

Melt the margarine in a skillet. Add the coconut and pecans, and cook until golden brown, stirring frequently. Remove from the heat. Beat the puréed sweet potatoes, cream cheese, and condensed milk in the bowl of an electric mixer until smooth. Fold in the thawed whipped topping. Spread one-fourth of the cream cheese mixture in each pie shell. Drizzle one-fourth of the caramel topping on top of the cream cheese mixture. Sprinkle one-fourth of each coconut and pecan mixture on top of the caramel topping. Repeat the layers three times. Cover and freeze until firm.

Let stand at room temperature for 5 minutes before serving.

MAKES 6 TO 8 SERVINGS

Apple Sweet Potato Squares

ingredients

1 16-ounce can sweet potatoes,
  drained

½ cup firmly packed brown sugar

3 eggs

½ teaspoon cinnamon

¼ teaspoon freshly grated nutmeg

¼ cup margarine, softened

2 cups packaged biscuit mix

1 cup chopped and peeled
  tart apples

⅓ cup raisins

¼ cup chopped pecans

Glaze

¾ cup confectioners' sugar

2 tablespoons orange juice

Preheat the oven to 350°. Spray a 13x9-inch glass baking dish with nonstick vegetable spray. Purée the sweet potatoes in a food processor. Cream the brown sugar and eggs together in a large bowl. Add the cinnamon, nutmeg, and margarine, beating well. Add the biscuit mix, and mix well. Fold in the apples, raisins, pecans, and puréed sweet potatoes. Pour into the prepared baking dish and spread evenly. Bake for 30 minutes or until done.

To make the Glaze

Combine the confectioners' sugar and orange juice in a small bowl.

Drizzle the glaze over the cooled cake. Cut into 2x3-inch squares.

MAKES 15 SQUARES

Sweet Potato Custard Pie

ingredients

1¼ cups puréed, canned sweet
  potatoes

2 large egg yolks

2 large whole eggs

1 cup whole milk

½ cup heavy cream

¼ cup firmly packed brown sugar

¼ cup sugar

½ teaspoon vanilla extract

¼ teaspoon freshly grated nutmeg

1 baked 9-inch pie shell

Preheat the oven to 350°. Blend together the sweet potatoes, egg yolks, whole eggs, milk, cream, sugars, vanilla, and nutmeg in a large bowl. Pour into the baked pie shell. Bake for 40 to 45 minutes or until a knife inserted in the center comes out clean. Allow to cool before serving.

MAKES 6 TO 8 SERVINGS

Sweet Potato Tassies

ingredients

Crust

2 3-ounce packages cream cheese, softened

1 cup all-purpose flour, sifted

½ cup margarine or butter

Filling

1½ cups cooked, puréed sweet potatoes

1 egg, beaten

1 tablespoon salted butter, softened

1 teaspoon vanilla extract

⅓ cup firmly packed brown sugar

¼ cup finely chopped pecans (optional)

Combine the cream cheese, flour, and margarine in a large bowl and mix until a dough forms. Cover and refrigerate for at least 2 hours.

Pinch off small pieces of chilled dough and roll into 1-inch balls. Place each ball in the center of a 1¾-inch miniature muffin cup. With your thumb, press the dough against the bottom and sides of the muffin cups, forming a tart shell. Remove only part of the dough at a time from the refrigerator to work on and keep the remaining dough chilled. The dough becomes too sticky to shape at room temperature.

To make the Filling

Preheat the oven to 325°. Mix the sweet potatoes, beaten egg, butter, vanilla, and brown sugar together in a medium bowl. Fill each tassie three-fourths full. Bake for 25 to 30 minutes. Cool on a cake rack.

To remove the cake, run a knife around the edges and lift out.

The finely chopped pecans may be used for a firmer tassie. You may have some filling left over.

MAKES 48 MINIATURE TASSIES

Sweet Potato Cream Cheese Pie

ingredients

2 cups graham cracker crumbs

2 tablespoons unsweetened
   applesauce

½ cup low-fat cream cheese

5 tablespoons maple syrup

1 tablespoon honey

¼ cup fresh orange juice

1 tablespoon cinnamon

¼ teaspoon nutmeg

¼ teaspoon cloves

¼ teaspoon allspice

¼ teaspoon ginger

2 tablespoons vanilla extract

3 cups baked, peeled, and mashed
   sweet potatoes

1 egg

2 egg whites

Preheat oven to 350°. Lightly spray a 9-inch pie pan with nonstick vegetable coating. Combine graham cracker crumbs and applesauce in processor and pulse until mixture is combined. Press in pie pan to make crust. Set aside.

Cream low-fat cream cheese, maple syrup, honey, orange juice, spices, and vanilla in a food processor. Add sweet potato and blend until smooth. Add egg and egg whites one at a time and blend until smooth.

Pour filling into crust and smooth top with a spatula. Bake 45 to 50 minutes until top of pie is set and no longer sticky to the touch. Cool on wire rack and refrigerate.

MAKES 12 SERVINGS, EACH CONTAINING APPROXIMATELY: 165 CALORIES, 29 GM. CARBOHYDRATE, 3 GM. FAT, 24 GM. CHOLESTEROL, 4 GM. PROTEIN, 163 MG. SODIUM, 2 GM. FIBER

—*from* Great Tastes: Healthy Living from Canyon Ranch

The Pirates' House
Sweet Potato Soufflé

ingredients

1 29-ounce can sweet potatoes

⅔ cup sugar

¼ cup margarine or butter

1 egg

½ cup orange juice

½ cup pineapple juice

1 teaspoon vanilla

1 8-ounce can crushed pineapple,
    drained, reserve juice

1 apple, chopped fine

¼ cup chopped pecans

1 cup or more miniature
    marshmallows

Preheat the oven to 350°. Butter a 1-quart casserole dish. Beat the sweet potatoes until smooth in the bowl of an electric mixer. Beat in the sugar, margarine, egg, orange juice, pineapple juice, and vanilla, blending well after each addition. Stir in the pineapple, apple, and pecans. Pour into the prepared dish and top with marshmallows. Bake about 20 to 25 minutes until the marshmallows are brown.

MAKES 6 TO 8 SERVINGS

The Pirates' House Restaurant located in Savannah, Georgia is a must-do for every Savannah visitor. This historic building was one of my children's favorite places to eat during our visits. In addition to this marvelous soufflé, they serve many other traditional-style Southern dishes.

Sweet Potato Lace Cups or Top Hats

ingredients

1 medium sweet potato

Peanut oil

Wash and peel the sweet potato. Shred like spaghetti in a food processor. Pour enough peanut oil into a skillet to coat the bottom. Heat the oil. Add a portion of the shredded sweet potato and quickly fry in a thin layer the size and shape of a lace cookie until crisp.

MAKES 6 TO 8 LACE CUPS OR TOP HATS

These lace cups or top hats are ideal for a custard of any flavor. They are also useful when creating desserts that stack or layer such as crepes. Top hats make interesting toppings on cheesecakes or other desserts. I have even used these as a lining for an individual slice of pork tenderloin for a delicious and colorful presentation.

Sweet Potato
friendship recipes

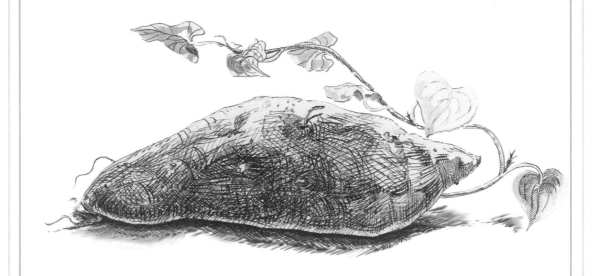

Just as I have a Friendship Garden for all the cuttings and pass-a-long plants from friends and relatives, I have a collection of Friendship Recipes from my friends who are also great hostesses and set a fine table.

Judy Gray, a neighbor and sorority sister of mine, shared several sweet potato recipes with me that she frequently uses at her many lovely dinner parties.

Thanksgiving Sweet Potatoes with Oatmeal Topping

ingredients

7 large sweet potatoes (about 5 pounds)

¼ cup butter, unsalted and softened

2 teaspoons salt

¼ cup firmly packed brown sugar

¼ cup orange juice

¼ cup orange marmalade

1 tablespoon finely grated peeled ginger root

Topping

3 cups crisp oatmeal cookie crumbs

6 tablespoons cold unsalted butter, sliced

Boil the sweet potatoes in a large pot in water to cover until tender. Peel and purée in a food processor. Add ¼ cup of butter, salt, and brown sugar, and pulse until blended. Combine the sweet potato mixture, orange juice, marmalade, and ginger root in a large bowl, stirring well. Spray a 13x9-inch baking dish with nonstick vegetable spray. Spread the mixture evenly in the pan. This may be made the day before, covered, and refrigerated. Bring the potato mixture to room temperature before proceeding.

To make the Topping

Grind the cookies into fine crumbs in a food processor. Add 6 tablespoons of butter and pulse until the mixture resembles cookie dough. Cover and chill until firm. The topping may also be made the day before and refrigerated.

Preheat the oven to 400°. Crumble the topping over the potato mixture. Bake in the middle of the oven for about 20 minutes or until the topping is brown.

MAKES 8 TO 10 SERVINGS

Judy's Pralines and Sweet Potatoes

ingredients

2 16-ounce cans sweet potatoes,
   drained and mashed
1 cup heavy cream
½ cup margarine, melted
1 teaspoon salt
2 cups sugar
4 eggs
½ cup sweet sherry

Topping

2 cups firmly packed brown sugar
1 cup all-purpose flour
½ cup margarine, melted
2 cups English walnut pieces

Preheat the oven to 350°. Combine the sweet potatoes, cream, margarine, salt, sugar, eggs, and sherry in a large bowl, blending well after each addition. Spray a 1-quart casserole with nonstick vegetable spray. Pour the mixture into the dish.

To make the Topping

Blend the sugar, flour, and melted margarine together in a small bowl. Stir in the English walnuts.

Sprinkle the nuts over the top of the sweet potato mixture. Bake for 45 minutes.

Maple Syrup Apples and Sweet Potatoes

ingredients

4 medium sweet potatoes

6 tart green apples

2 tablespoons lemon juice

¼ cup apple cider

¾ cup maple syrup

½ teaspoon salt

¼ cup unsalted butter or margarine

Preheat the oven to 375°. Spray a 13x9-inch glass baking dish with nonstick vegetable spray. Wash and peel the sweet potatoes. Slice the sweet potatoes crosswise into ¼-inch pieces. Cover with cold water until the apples are prepared. Wash the apples, peel, core, and slice into ¼-inch pieces. Sprinkle with lemon juice. Layer the sweet potatoes and apples, alternating in rows. Combine the apple cider, maple syrup, salt, and butter in a saucepan and bring to a boil. Pour over the sweet potatoes and apples. Cover the dish with aluminum foil and bake for 1 hour.

Uncover the casserole. Reduce the heat to 350° and bake until the sweet potatoes and apples are done and the syrup is a thick glaze. Serve hot.

MAKES 6 TO 8 SERVINGS

Sara Deitch has four sons, one of whom is a classmate of my son, Rob. Sara is always serving huge family meals and including Rob, as well as others, to dine with them. It is a coveted invitation for Rob, as he knows that there will be good company, excellent food, and superior conversation. One of her specialties is this New England-style sweet potato dish flavored with maple syrup.

Sweet Potatoes in Apricot Sauce

ingredients

3 pounds sweet potatoes

1 cup firmly packed brown sugar

1½ tablespoons cornstarch

¼ teaspoon salt

⅛ teaspoon cinnamon

½ cup hot water

2 teaspoons orange rind

1 cup apricot nectar

2 tablespoons margarine or butter

½ cup raisins or pecans

Preheat the oven to 350°. Boil the sweet potatoes in a large pot in water to cover until tender. Drain and cool. Peel and cut in half lengthwise. Place in a 2-quart casserole. Combine the brown sugar, cornstarch, salt, and cinnamon in a saucepan. Add the water, orange rind, and apricot nectar, and bring to a boil, stirring constantly. Remove from the heat and stir in the butter and raisins or pecans. Pour over the potatoes. Bake for 25 minutes.

Tatties An' Tatties

ingredients

3 medium sweet potatoes

4 medium white potatoes

2 tablespoons unsalted butter

Salt and freshly ground white
   pepper to taste

Scrub the sweet potatoes and white potatoes. Cover the potatoes with water and boil until tender in a large pot. Drain and cool. Peel both the sweet potatoes and white potatoes. Mash with a potato masher or pulse in a food processor. Add the butter, salt, and freshly ground white pepper.

Pat Walsh serves this adaptation of an old Scottish dish called Tatties an' Neeps (turnips and potatoes). I always served Tatties an' Neeps at the annual Robert Burns Birthday Dinner. Pat's version is a mixture of mashed sweet potatoes and mashed white potatoes, and it is absolutely delicious.

Orange Sweet Potatoes

ingredients

6 sweet potatoes

3 navel oranges, peeled and thinly
  sliced

¾ cup sugar

½ cup butter, melted

1 cup orange juice

2 tablespoons lemon juice

Preheat the oven to 375°. Spray a 1-quart casserole dish with butter spray. Boil the sweet potatoes in a large pot in water to cover until tender, or bake for 1 hour and 30 minutes until done. Baking gives them a sweeter flavor.

Cool, peel, and slice the sweet potatoes very thin. Place a single layer of sweet potatoes in the casserole dish. Add a layer of orange slices. Brush with butter and sprinkle the sugar over. Continue layering, ending with a layer of sweet potatoes, butter, and sugar (about 3 layers). Mix the orange juice with the lemon juice in a small bowl and pour over the potatoes. Bake for about 1 hour and 30 minutes or until a syrup has formed and the top is tinged brown.

MAKES 6 TO 8 SERVINGS

My children and I have shared Christmas holidays with my good friend Nancy Carter Thompson from Augusta, Georgia. This is the dish she prepares for Christmas dinner and is a favorite of her husband, Mason, and son, Scott.

Kentucky Bourbon Sweet Potatoes

ingredients

2 16-ounce cans sweet potatoes

1 tablespoon brown sugar (or more
  to taste)

¼ cup frozen orange juice
  concentrate

¼ cup bourbon (or more to taste)

1 cup pecan pieces

Preheat the oven to 350°. Spray a 1-quart casserole with nonstick vegetable spray. Drain and mash the sweet potatoes. Add the brown sugar, orange juice concentrate, and bourbon, blending well. Spread the sweet potato mixture evenly in the dish. Sprinkle with pecan pieces.

Bake in the center of the oven for 30 minutes.

Nancy Thompson's mother, Madeline Carter, always serves this dish for her holiday entertaining in Kentucky.

Covered Dish Soufflé Crunch

ingredients

3 large sweet potatoes

3 eggs, separated

½ cup milk

¼ teaspoon salt

1 tablespoon vanilla extract

3 tablespoons butter

1 cup sugar

Crunch Topping

3 tablespoons butter

½ cup self-rising flour

1 cup firmly packed brown sugar

1 cup chopped pecans or walnuts

Preheat the oven to 325°. Spray a 1-quart soufflé dish with nonstick butter spray. Boil the sweet potatoes in a large pot in water to cover until tender. Drain, cool, peel, and purée in a food processor. Separate the eggs and add the egg yolks, milk, salt, and vanilla to the sweet potatoes. Cream 3 tablespoons of butter and the sugar together in a medium bowl. Add the creamed mixture to the sweet potato mixture. Beat the egg whites until they stand in a stiff peak. Fold into the sweet potato mixture. Pour the mixture into the prepared dish, smoothing the top.

To make the Topping

Combine 3 tablespoons of butter, the flour, brown sugar, and pecans in a medium bowl and mix together with a pastry cutter. Spread over the sweet potato mixture. Bake for about 30 minutes in the center of the oven.

MAKES 6 TO 8 SERVINGS

Certain types of dishes have a special place in my Friendship Recipe file—the dishes that make great "covered dish" gifts to friends and neighbors for illness, moving, or any situation that begs for a prepared food contribution.

The Covered Dish Soufflé Crunch is the dish I make most often for friends, and they have come to expect it. It is a great dish to prepare ahead. To freeze or make the day before, do not separate the eggs. Just add them beaten together. The soufflé will not be as light.

Madeleine's Thanksgiving Sweet Potato Casserole

ingredients

6 to 8 small sweet potatoes

1 6-ounce can frozen orange juice

½ to 1 cup butter, melted

1 teaspoon ginger

1 tablespoon cinnamon

½ teaspoon coriander

¼ teaspoon mace

¼ teaspoon cloves

¼ teaspoon cayenne pepper

½ cup raisins

2 cups black walnut halves

1 bag large marshmallows

Preheat the oven to 350°. Scrub the sweet potatoes and spray with nonstick vegetable spray. Place on a cookie sheet and bake for about 1 hour or until caramelized.

Cool and peel the sweet potatoes. Chop into chunks for easier handling. Mash the sweet potatoes in a large bowl until there are very few pea-size pieces. Add the orange juice and melted butter, and stir. Combine the ginger, cinnamon, coriander, mace, cloves, and cayenne pepper in a small glass dish, and mix together. Add the spices to the sweet potato mixture and stir well. This mixture may be stored covered in the refrigerator for 2 to 3 days. On the day of serving the casserole, bring the sweet potato mixture to room temperature. Preheat the oven to 350°. Add the raisins and walnuts and stir well. Spray the casserole dish with nonstick vegetable spray. Spoon the mixture into the casserole, smoothing the surface flat. Top with marshmallows. Stagger the rows with a ¼-inch space between each one. Fill in the remaining spaces with walnut pieces if desired. Bake for about 30 minutes or until the marshmallows are melted and brown on top.

My good friend Madeleine Watt, a talented artist and illustrator of this book, shares a recipe that reflects her childhood in both Hepsibah, Georgia, and Austin, Texas. This is a traditional Georgia holiday dish with a touch of Central Texas thrown in for an extra sparkle.

Sweet Potato Hush Puppies

ingredients

1 16-ounce can sweet potatoes

2 tablespoons self-rising cornmeal

2 tablespoons all-purpose flour

2 tablespoons honey

Milk

2 tablespoons vegetable oil

Drain and mash the sweet potatoes. Add the cornmeal, flour, and honey to the sweet potatoes. Add enough milk to the mixture to moisten until the consistency of cookie dough.

Drop by spoonfuls into hot vegetable oil. Fry until a crispy brown.

MAKES 6 SERVINGS

My mother, Idella North, of Hahira, Georgia, is the most efficient cook I've ever witnessed, including professional cooks. From planning and organizing to the execution of all meals, not a movement is wasted or repeated. She plans days ahead and can multiply whatever is being served to accommodate last-minute guests or relatives who, knowing they are always welcome, feel free to drop in at serving time. My mother grew up in a family of eleven children where everyone had a household responsibility. Later, when she had five children and a household of her own to run, she utilized the culinary skills which she acquired as a child. Everyone has always marveled at how quickly she works and of course my mother has always been amazed at how some folks could make meal preparation into a full day. Her philosophy was always to "get done what you had to do to keep the program going so that you had time to do the things that were fun." Of course, Mother asked me not to use her name in my cookbook, which is so typical, as she says these sweet potato recipes are dishes that have been done forever.

Karen North's Nutty Sweet Potato Biscuits

ingredients

2 cups sweet potatoes, mashed

¾ cup sugar

½ cup butter or margarine

1 teaspoon vanilla extract

2¾ cup all-purpose flour

4 teaspoons baking powder

1¼ teaspoons salt

½ teaspoon cinnamon

½ teaspoon freshly grated nutmeg

¾ cup finely chopped pecans

Boil the sweet potatoes in a large pot in water to cover until tender. Drain, cook, peel, and blend in a food processor. Add the sugar, butter, and vanilla to the sweet potato mixture, blending well in the food processor. Sift together the flour, baking powder, salt, cinnamon, and nutmeg in a large bowl. Add the flour mixture to the sweet potato mixture, ⅓ cup at a time, and pulse. Remove and stir in the finely chopped pecans (these could be chopped in the food processor with the French blade).

Preheat the oven to 450°. Turn the mixture onto a floured pastry cloth. Knead lightly. Roll dough into ½-inch thickness. Cut with a biscuit cutter and place on a lightly greased baking sheet. Bake for 12 minutes or until brown.

MAKES 18 BISCUITS

Mother's biscuits are famous. Since I was a toddler I remember relatives, friends of relatives, neighbors, church members, etc., asking Mother to teach them how to make biscuits. I have tried all my life to make those biscuits and finally gave up a few years ago. When mother asked what my son, Rob, would like as a special treat when he visited or for a birthday gift, it was always "Gamma's biscuits, please." This is not Mother's recipe for those impossible-to-duplicate biscuits, but for another that I and others can make very easily and successfully.

Mother's Sweet Potato Puff

ingredients

4 cups canned sweet potatoes

2 tablespoons sherry

2 tablespoons firmly packed
   brown sugar

¾ cup cream

1 tablespoon butter

¼ teaspoon freshly ground nutmeg

½ teaspoon salt

2 egg yolks, beaten

2 egg whites, whipped

Preheat the oven to 425°. Spray a casserole dish with nonstick vegetable spray. Drain the sweet potatoes and mash in a food processor. Blend in the sherry, brown sugar, cream, butter, nutmeg, salt, and egg yolks. Fold in the whipped egg whites. Pour the sweet potato mixture into the dish. Bake for 15 to 20 minutes.

MAKES 6 TO 8 SERVINGS

Sweet Potatoes
around the world

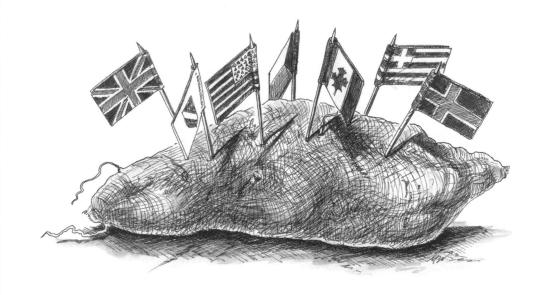

GREAT BRITAIN
Sweet Potato Rock Cakes

ingredients

2 cups sweet potatoes, drained

2 eggs

¾ cup firmly packed brown sugar

½ cup butter, softened

1½ cups all-purpose flour, sifted

¼ teaspoon baking powder

½ teaspoon baking soda

⅛ teaspoon salt

½ teaspoon cinnamon

¼ teaspoon allspice

½ teaspoon ground cloves

¼ cup orange juice or sherry

¾ cup chopped dates

¼ cup chopped walnuts *pecans*

¾ cup citron

Preheat the oven to 375°. Spray a cookie sheet with vegetable spray. Purée the drained sweet potatoes in a food processor. Add the eggs one at a time, using the pulse on the food processor. Add the brown sugar and softened butter, and process until creamy. Sift together the flour, baking powder, soda, salt, cinnamon, allspice, and cloves in a medium bowl. Add the dry ingredients and orange juice or sherry to the sweet potato mixture alternating in two parts each. Beat until smooth. Stir in the dates, walnuts, and citron. Drop the rock cakes by heaping teaspoonful onto the cookie sheet. Bake for 12 to 15 minutes.

These delicious rock cakes may be stored in an airtight tin.

Although sweet potatoes are not served in the British Isles very much, rock cakes are a very British dish. My son's wife, Clio, makes great rock cakes.

ITALY
Risotto Sweet Potatoes

ingredients

2 medium sweet potatoes

Tarragon leaves, chopped

1 tablespoon olive oil

1 sweet onion, peeled and chopped

2 garlic cloves, peeled and minced

2 cups Italian rice, arborio or pearl

1 cup peeled and thinly sliced
  carrots

1 red pepper, seeded and chopped

1 yellow pepper, seeded and
  chopped

1 green pepper, seeded and
  chopped

½ teaspoon salt

Freshly ground white pepper

5 cups water

Wash and peel the sweet potatoes. Slice crosswise in ⅛-inch slices. Place the sweet potatoes in a microwave-safe dish. Add ¼ cup water and sprinkle with tarragon leaves. Cover and microwave on high for 2 minutes.

Heat the olive oil in a large skillet. Sauté the onion and garlic for 5 minutes. Add the sweet potatoes, risotto, carrots, peppers, salt, pepper, and half the water. Cover and cook on medium heat for about 10 minutes, stirring occasionally. Add the remaining water, lower the heat, and cook for 10 minutes, stirring frequently. Remove from the heat and cover.

MAKES 6 TO 8 SERVINGS

JAPAN

My friend Virginia Stippes Anami told me this wonderful sweet potato story at a dinner party about how important sweet potatoes are to Japanese food culture. "The sellers go up and down the streets in the winter time in a small open truck with the potatoes roasting over charcoal heated hot stones." (In the past the roasted sweet potatoes were sold from a cart.)

The ditty they sing goes like this:

"Yaki imo, Yaki imo, Ishi Yaki imo.

Benkyo shinai ko ni uranai zo.

Yaki imo, Yaki imo, Ishi Yaki imo."

Translation:

"Roasted Sweet Potatoes, Roasted Sweet Potatoes, Roasted over Hot Stones,

But I won't sell them to kids who aren't studying hard, Roasted Sweet Potatoes,

Roasted Sweet Potatoes, Roasted over Hot Stones."

These potatoes are called *satsumaimo*. That is, potatoes of Satsuma, the old district name of southern Kyushu, now the prefecture of Kagoshima, the sister state for Georgia. The most famous sweet potato recipe in Japan is eaten on the New Year and is called kinton. It is a gooey sweet mass mixed with chestnuts and served in a lacquer box with bitter tea. This kinton recipe is from Ginny's husband's sister, Kimiko.

Kimiko's Kinton

ingredients

3 sweet potatoes

Gardenia plant seeds

2 cups sugar

3 tablespoons honey

2 tablespoons mirin (sweetened sake)

1 cup sweet chestnuts, drained

Wash and peel the sweet potatoes. Cut in large lengthwise slabs and soak in water. Boil or steam until tender. Purée or mash and push through a strainer. Stir in a few gardenia plant seeds to add a golden color. Place the strained sweet potatoes in a heavy saucepan with sugar, honey, and mirin. Cook over medium heat until a sticky consistency and the texture of soft mashed potatoes. Add the drained sweet chestnuts and serve.

MAKES 4 TO 6 SERVINGS

JAPAN
Tempura Sweet Potatoes

ingredients

6 medium sweet potatoes

1 cup ice water

1 egg

¾ cup all-purpose flour

1 teaspoon salt

⅛ teaspoon baking soda

2 cups vegetable oil

Soy sauce

Wash and peel the sweet potatoes. Cut the sweet potatoes in half lengthwise and then cut into 1/4-inch slices. Beat the ice water with the egg in a mixing bowl on high setting until frothy. Add the flour, salt, and baking soda and mix on low setting until all moistened and blended. Dip 6 to 8 pieces of the sweet potato into the batter and fry them in a hot skillet of vegetable oil, turning them once, about 2 minutes until golden brown. Lift with a slotted spoon and place on several layers of paper towel to absorb the grease. Discard greasy paper towels and place on fresh paper towels on a cookie sheet. Keep warm in the oven at 200° until time to serve. Continue frying the remaining sweet potato slices. Serve with soy sauce.

MAKES 6 SERVINGS

This is a very popular Japanese sweet potato dish. Tempura was introduced to Japan by the seafaring Portuguese several hundred years ago.

CHINA
Chaozhou Youguo

ingredients

2 cups mashed sweet potatoes

Red bean paste to taste

Cornstarch

Peanut oil

Pureé the sweet potatoes in a food processor and add red bean paste to taste. Form into balls and roll in cornstarch. Drop one by one into a skillet of very hot peanut oil and fry to a golden brown nugget.

This dish was served by the Ministry of Culture to my friend Virginia Stippes Anami on her recent visit to Beijing. The chef was eighty years old, and this is one of his specialties.

CHINA
Baixu

ingredients

Sweet potatoes
Oil

Wash the sweet potatoes and rub with cooking oil. Wrap in foil and place over coals or around the edges. Roast until tender, turning once.

Baixu is pronounced bye-shoo. It is simply roasted sweet potatoes. In China they are sold by vendors pushing carts around the cities in the winter, particularly up north. They are roasted over hot coals and are sometimes sold by vendors who have set up oil drums with coals. They are served in the skins and eaten out of the sweet potato jacket.

CHINA
Canton Sweet Potato Balls

ingredients

3 medium sweet potatoes

2 tablespoons sugar

½ cup all-purpose flour

Peanut oil

Peel and quarter the sweet potatoes. Place in a pan and cover with water to simmer about 30 minutes until soft. Drain and mash the sweet potatoes and mix with the sugar. Sift the flour and gradually add to the mixture, mixing thoroughly. Dust hands with flour and roll the mixture into 1½-inch balls. Deep fry the balls in 350° oil about 2 to 3 minutes until golden brown.

PHILIPPINES
Fish Soup

ingredients

1 medium sweet potato

6 cups water

2 onions, finely chopped

3 large tomatoes, chopped

1⅓ cups chopped frozen spinach

2 teaspoons finely grated
   lemon rind

1 tablespoon tamarind pulp

Salt and pepper to taste

1½ pound white fish fillets,
   chopped

Lemon slices for garnish

Wash the sweet potato. Boil the sweet potato in a large pot in water to cover for about 15 minutes until tender. Drain and cool. Peel and slice into 1-inch pieces.

Combine 6 cups of water, onions, tomatoes, spinach, lemon rind, and tamarind in a stock pot. Season with salt and pepper. Bring to a boil. Reduce the heat and simmer for 15 minutes.

Stir in the chopped fish fillets and simmer for 15 minutes more. Garnish with lemon slices.

MAKES 6 SERVINGS

WEST AFRICA
Fufu

ingredients

4 medium sweet potatoes
Salt

Wash the sweet potatoes and boil about 30 minutes until tender. Drain, peel, and purée the sweet potatoes. Add the salt. Purée again until it is a paste. (In West Africa, this is done with a pestle.) Wet hands and roll into bite-size balls. Spray or sprinkle with water to keep moist. Cover tightly. Serve with soups and stews.

AFRICA
African Yam Soup

ingredients

2 teaspoons vegetable oil

1 large onion, peeled and chopped

2 small hot chilies, seeded and chopped

2 medium tomatoes, peeled, seeded, and chopped

1 pound sweet potatoes or yams, peeled and cubed

2 cups beef broth

1 cup water

¼ teaspoon salt

Freshly ground white pepper

2 tablespoons chopped fresh parsley for garnish

Heat the oil in a stock pot and sauté the onion until translucent. Add the chilies and tomatoes, and cook for about 5 minutes. Add the sweet potatoes, broth, and water. Bring the soup to a boil, reduce the heat, and simmer for 20 to 30 minutes until the sweet potatoes are soft.

Purée the soup in a blender. Return the purée to the pan. Add the salt and pepper and heat thoroughly. Garnish with parsley.

MAKES 4 TO 6 SERVINGS

BRAZIL
Brazilian Sweet Potato Soup

ingredients

1 29-ounce can sweet potatoes, drained
4 tablespoons butter
¾ cup finely chopped onions
4 cups cold water
½ bunch parsley, chopped
1 teaspoon salt
Freshly ground white pepper
½ teaspoon orange zest
⅛ teaspoon mace
2 tablespoons cornstarch
3 cups milk
½ cup chopped peanuts

Purée the sweet potatoes in a food processor. Melt the butter in a stock pot and sauté the onions until tender. Add the water, sweet potatoes, parsley, salt, and pepper. Cover and bring to a boil. Reduce the heat and simmer for 30 minutes.

Pour the soup into a food processor and purée the solids. Return to the stock pot and add the orange zest and mace. Blend the cornstarch into a small amount of milk and then blend in the remaining milk. Pour the milk mixture into the soup and mix well.

Serve with chopped peanuts on top.

MAKES 6 TO 8 SERVINGS

ARGENTINA
Latin Sweet Potato Soup

ingredients

2 large sweet potatoes

4 tablespoons butter

2 cups finely chopped onion

2 cloves garlic, peeled and mashed

¼ teaspoon thyme

1 leek, trimmed, cleaned, and
   chopped

⅛ teaspoon freshly grated nutmeg

2½ cups chicken broth

½ cup half and half

Salt to taste

½ cup sour cream or Crème
   Fraîche (see page 26)

2 green onions, sliced

4 tablespoons packaged Adobo
   sauce (available in most
   supermarkets)

Boil the sweet potatoes in a large pot in water to cover until slightly tender. Drain, cool, peel, and purée. Melt the butter in a saucepan and sauté the onion, garlic, thyme, and leek until tender. Add the freshly grated nutmeg and the chicken broth. Whisk the puréed sweet potatoes into the mixture and reduce the heat. Stir in the half and half. Season with salt.

To serve, place a spoon of sour cream or Crème Fraîche into each bowl and sprinkle with green onions and Adobo sauce.

THE CARIBBEAN
Sweet Potato Fritters

ingredients

3 medium sweet potatoes

2 eggs

2 tablespoons margarine

Kosher salt

Freshly ground white pepper

½ cup wheat germ

All-purpose flour

Olive oil

Wash the sweet potatoes and cover with cold water. Bring to a boil and cook about 30 minutes until tender. Drain, cool, peel, and purée in a food processor. Add the eggs, margarine, salt, and pepper and beat until smooth. Shape into bite-size patties. Coat with flour and wheat germ. Chill until firm. Fry in hot oil until golden brown.

MOROCCO
Sweet Potatoes with Cumin and Onions

ingredients

3 tablespoons unsalted butter

1 medium onion, chopped

1½ tablespoons cumin seeds

2 medium sweet potatoes, cooked

Melt the butter in a heavy skillet and sauté the onions over medium heat about 5 minutes until softened. Remove the onions and add the cumin seeds to the hot skillet. Lightly roast (about 1 to 2 minutes) until fragrant.

Slice the cooked sweet potatoes into ½-inch pieces and add to hot skillet with the cumin seeds and onions. Stir together and cook about 5 to 8 minutes until the potatoes are slightly browned.

MAKES 6 SERVINGS

PORTUGAL
Sweet Potato Dessert

ingredients

1 medium sweet potato

⅔ cup sugar

⅓ cup water

8 egg yolks

Nutmeg, freshly grated

½ cup whipping cream

Wash the sweet potato. Boil the sweet potato in a large pot in water to cover until tender. Cool and peel. Purée the sweet potato in a food processor. Heat the sugar and ⅓ cup water in a saucepan over low heat, stirring constantly, until the mixture forms a syrup. Add the sweet potato purée and continue to cook over low heat for about 5 minutes. Remove from the heat and cool to lukewarm.

Add the egg yolks, one at a time, beating well after each addition. Cook again over low heat until thick, creamy, and the mixture will part when you cut it with a spoon or spatula. Remove from the heat and add nutmeg to taste. Immerse the pan in a pot of ice water to cool. Divide among 6 parfait glasses or sherbet stems and chill.

Top with whipped cream and more freshly grated nutmeg before serving.

MAKES 6 SERVINGS

Great to do the day before a party.

MEXICO
Camote

ingredients

4 medium sweet potatoes

1½ cups firmly packed brown sugar

¾ cup water

3 tablespoons butter

¼ teaspoon salt

Wash and peel the sweet potatoes. Cut into 4 pieces lengthwise. Combine the brown sugar, water, and butter in a heavy saucepan, and bring to a boil. Reduce the heat and add the sweet potatoes and salt. Simmer until the sweet potatoes are soft. Remove from the heat and cool.

Place the sweet potatoes on a cake rack to dry. Chill before serving.

MAKES 6 SERVINGS

TURKEY
Halva

ingredients

1½ cups canned sweet potatoes, drained

4 tablespoons butter

1 cup milk

1 14-ounce can sweetened condensed milk

¼ cup honey

½ cup firmly packed brown sugar

2 tablespoons rose water

1 teaspoon ground cardamon

1 cup pistachio nuts or ½ cup sesame seeds

Purée the sweet potatoes in a food processor. Combine the butter, milk, sweetened condensed milk, honey, and brown sugar in a heavy saucepan. Cook slowly over low heat, stirring continuously, until the mixture reaches a soft ball when a small amount is dropped in a cup of cold water. Remove from the heat and add the puréed sweet potatoes.

Cook again slowly for 5 minutes. Remove from the heat and add the rose water, cardamon, and nuts or seeds, and mix thoroughly.

Spray a glass baking dish with nonstick spray. Pour the sweet potato mixture into the prepared dish. Press down and chill to set.

MAKES 8 TO 10 SERVINGS

Index

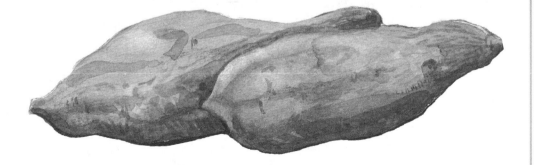